GETTING OLDER...IT'S AVOIDABLE!

GETTING OLDER...IT'S AVOIDABLE!

THE STRATEGY TO KEEP THE YOUTH OF YOUR CELLS AND YOUR BODY

DANIEL MINIER

WALK TO

COPYRIGHT © 2017 DANIEL MINIER

All rights reserved.

GETTING OLDER...IT'S AVOIDABLE!

The Strategy to Keep the Youth of Your Cells and Your Body

ISBN   978-1-5445-0054-6 *Paperback*

  978-1-5445-0055-3 *Ebook*

Maintaining the health of our youth for the rest of our lives is a lifelong task.

CONTENTS

———

WHY I WROTE THIS BOOK

· 1 ·

THE PROBLEM

———

In our industrialized society, we benefit from an increasingly longer life expectancy, but the additional years of life we are given are accompanied by health problems that spoil our quality of life. **These health problems are avoidable**, and it is up to us to protect our health and that of our children in anticipation of a life expectancy that may reach 90 or even 100 years.

· 2 ·

THE SOLUTION

——

Scientific research in recent years and even in recent months has enabled us to understand that the aging of the body, age-related diseases, and cancers are the result of the same process. These discoveries also let us determine targets we can act on and identify simple, effective tools to generally counteract the aging process.

WHY I WROTE THIS BOOK

· 3 ·

THE OBSTACLE

———

As health professionals, we wait for major clinical studies before taking action. Such studies take decades before providing reliable conclusions. So neither health professionals nor the authorities are inclined to take a lead in solving this major problem.

WHY I WROTE THIS BOOK

· 4 ·

THE THESIS

———

Waiting years for the conclusions of major clinical studies will mean the sacrifice of yet another generation. That is an awfully high price to pay, in terms of both money and quality of life.

The best approach, as presented in this book, is to pool the information from many hundreds of recent studies so we can understand how our bodies age. This knowledge will allow us, right now, to select targets and identify the best tools for maintaining our quality of life in the long term. That will enable us to protect our children's generation from useless aging and equip them to face its challenges.

INTRODUCTION

"Enjoy life while you're young, Dr. Minier! Things change as you get older." Hearing such advice from well-intentioned patients as they leave my office isn't a rare occurrence. And it resonates deeply because such statements are generally made by people living with aging-related discomforts. Such comments might seem mundane and could be considered as simply referring to an inevitable reality. But statements like these, which I hear every day in my office, should prompt us to take a closer look. What changes as you get older? And is the greatest consequence of aging being limited in the capacity to enjoy life?

Fortunately, the human characteristics of adaptability and resilience allow most people to grow older while maintaining a positive outlook, because they have acquired some wisdom. But as we know, while life expectancy is getting longer, health expectancy is stagnating; aging seems therefore to mean illness. But is there some portion of this aging process that could be considered "needless aging"? Is there something we could do to continue to enjoy life for longer, for much longer?

Fortunately, our knowledge about how the aging body works has grown greatly in recent years. Accordingly, in this book, we will be exploring strategies for remaining healthy as long as possible, even for our whole lives. We will begin by examining a key concept in understanding what is going on as the body ages. Then we will identify five targets that slow down *needless aging*. Some of these measures will seem instinctive, while others will be more surprising and may even appear counter to what society tells us are evolutionary successes. These approaches that we will be examining together have shown that they can have a real impact in scientific studies and, in addition, are easy to include our daily routines, as you will see. So let's get started!

CHAPTER 1

CONTEXT: OUR UNDERSTANDING OF HEALTH IS RAPIDLY EVOLVING

Aging is something new for humanity

A number of factors have contributed to improving life expectancy in the industrialized world: water purification, earlier detection of certain diseases, better medical care, and more sophisticated surgical techniques. The progress has been enormous: the life expectancy in industrialized countries rose from about 50 years in 1900 to about 80 in 2010. In the not-so-distant past, people died *young*; they didn't have time to grow older, to *age*. Gradually, our societies have started to expect a larger number of older people in the population, and that has let us observe and start to understand what goes on in the body at an advanced age.

Another statistic now presents a challenge for society: life expectancy with good health, also known as "health expectancy." In 2010, the health expectancy in the European Union was about 62 years...some 18 years shorter than the life expectancy of 80! More than a decade and a half during which people cannot enjoy their lives the way they used to. So what happens during those 15 or so years of life in poorer health?

The improvement in life expectancy has shed some light on certain diseases considered to be age-related such as cardiovascular diseases, degenerative joint diseases, neurological diseases of the Alzheimer's type, cancers, and deterioration in skin condition and bodily functions in general. These diseases only occur very rarely in young people. Because life expectancy in earlier centuries was shorter, ours are really the first generations to face these age-related diseases. These diseases are encountered more and more with an aging population, and we try to deal with them, but, as things stand, we are only reacting. So, we need to answer a crucial question: are these diseases that appear with age really part of a normal process?

And furthermore, could doctors intervene to keep us from "aging dangerously"?

Doctors facing an aging population

Consulting your doctor for early screening and having your health problems treated is an excellent way to improve your own life expectancy and your quality of life. But, as stated above, health expectancy hasn't really improved; people are living longer...with more and more health issues. This poses an initial problem for health-care systems: doctors devote more time than before to treating age-related diseases. As a result, they have become managers of disease and declining health, leaving them virtually no time to play their health-promotion role. Prevention falls increasingly by the wayside, so that people are deprived of the advice and motivation their doctor could provide.

"...health expectancy hasn't really improved; people are living longer but with more and more health issues."

The second problem results from the type of medicine practiced in our society. As doctors, we require solid clinical studies before making preventive recommendations. That's why we waited for major studies that lasted years before telling our patients to protect themselves from the sun to reduce the risk of skin cancers, to lower their salt intake to reduce hypertension, and to stop smoking to reduce the risk of certain cancers. As a result of the delays in making such recommendations, we have practically sacrificed a generation. It also means that if we had been more alert and more active in analyzing medical studies, we would have been able to offer better prevention on a number of levels. For example, in my specialty—dermatology—we would not have witnessed such an epidemic of skin cancers.

Waiting for major studies to issue recommendations offers several advantages for doctors and patients. For example, having solid clinical studies is normal and even essential before prescribing a medication that entails risks of side effects or generates additional costs for the patient or society. The great advantage of this approach is that we have medicine that is generally very reliable and safe. Its disadvantage is that when we acquire new knowledge about how the body works, we have to wait years before obtaining the results of clinical studies. Long-term studies are necessary to prevent just a single disease, so imagine how long such studies would take to verify impacts on long-term health and longevity. Do we have to wait for such results before acting?

"**Fortunately, our understanding of the processes that**

cause aging has clearly been growing quickly in recent years and even in recent months!"

There is no doubt that, one day, we will be able to benefit from the results of large-scale clinical studies. While waiting for them, however, what basis should we use to make wise choices to improve health expectancy? The lessons offered by a few centenarians are quite interesting, but they don't represent a solid enough foundation for their "tips" to be applied by the whole population. The supposedly extraordinary supplements sold by natural-product companies are too simplistic to prepare the body for healthy longevity. We must therefore look to other types of studies that seek to understand how the human body functions. Fortunately, our understanding of the processes that cause aging has clearly been growing quickly in recent years and even in recent months! Moreover, strategies to act on these processes are also better grounded. This allows us to act before official recommendations have been formulated, and we ought to do this to protect ourselves and our children against needless aging.

Why have we done nothing about aging?

First, because we are the first generations to have to deal with this scourge. Second—and this is another important part of the problem—during all the years that our bodies and cells suffer the damage that makes us age, during all those years when one cell starts on its evolution into a cancer, there aren't any symptoms. THE AGING PROCESS DOESN'T CAUSE ANY SYMPTOMS! Cancers, age-related diseases, and *needless aging* occur insidiously over a long time, and we only see a doctor when one such condition has reared its head.

For example, people consult a dermatologist when their skin has become fragile, when pigment spots have appeared, or when a skin cancer has been detected. These signs of premature aging have taken 15, 20, or even more years to form, and no symptoms were visible during that long period. The process is no different in other parts of the body. We consult a doctor when we are facing a fait accompli. Although certain approaches may partially reverse the situation, if we wait for the symptoms to occur before seeing a doctor, the only options available will be palliative.

"The *only* solution is, from an early age, to adopt lifestyle habits that will keep us "young" for a long time. For parents, this is a valuable legacy to leave to their children."

Aging: a responsibility for the individual...and for the family

Because the aging process occurs over many years and is asymptomatic, it is useless (and even reckless) to wait for symptoms to occur before taking action. The *only* solution is, from an early age, to adopt lifestyle habits that will keep us "young" for a long time. For parents, this is a valuable legacy to leave to their children. For each of us, as individuals responsible for our own health, it is never too late to adopt good habits. As shown in the following chapters, adopting certain strategies will enable us to limit *needless aging* and even reverse certain elements involved in cell aging.

CHAPTER 2

WE DON'T ALL AGE IN THE SAME WAY

———

What affects our chances of living a long time?

As we have seen, the treatment of infections, surgery, and the general improvement in health care have improved life expectancy. So, consulting your doctor for screening and early treatment of health conditions remains an excellent investment in a long life. But who, when encountering a very old person, hasn't wondered what their secret was. In talking to them, it is not unusual to learn that they are not the only ones in their family to attain very old age. Often, these families don't have any special secret: their asset is genes that favor longevity. Some people genetically have greater physical strength, others have greater intellectual abilities, and still others have longevity. If these genetically predisposed individuals are removed from the equation, however, it appears that genetics accounts for about 25% (and some authors propose even less than 10%) of the determinants of life expectancy. This leaves more than 75% for us to work on. This 75% is within our control and we are responsible for taking action. But is it worth investing in good habits? Will these "efforts" really allow us to maintain good health throughout life?

Can you get older without aging?

Those who claim that they have the secret of living until they are 150 years old are simply dealing in smoke and mirrors; nothing known now justifies such a claim. Life expectancy is genetically "limited" and human beings are not all equal in this respect. We must therefore—at least for now!—accept the reality of the situation. The purpose of this book is not to push back genetic boundaries. ITS OBJECTIVE IS REALISTIC AND ACHIEVABLE. Using the most relevant articles in the medical literature, we will be trying to reach our genetic limit, without losing function or with a minimum loss, and thereby maintain our physical and mental independence throughout our lifetimes. With a difference between health expectancy and life expectancy that can sometimes be as much as 15 years, it seems worth the effort. But is getting older without aging really possible?

My fellow dermatologists and I have front-row seats to witnessing that aging is not the same thing as getting old. Every day, we observe people's skin. The skin of some people is much older than that of others of the same age. And, on the same person, certain areas have aged more quickly than others. In some places, the skin is much more wrinkled, has undergone pigmentation changes, lost elasticity, and begun to present cancerous lesions, whereas, elsewhere, the color and texture have remained homogeneous and no precancerous tissue is present. I often call this difference to the attention of my patients. Have a look at your skin. Often, it is easy to see that it has not aged equally everywhere. Compare the skin on your face to that on your buttocks; the skin on the outside of your forearm to that on the inside. We know that these differences are caused by aging that has been accelerated by the sun. It's obvious: skin can age faster or slower... and it can get older without aging! Observing the skin offers a wonderful insight into aging: the same person will have skin that has aged in some locations but has a much younger appearance in others. So what must have happened *inside* this prematurely aged skin?

"Like our skin, our whole bodies can age faster or slower...and our whole bodies can also get older without aging."

Studies have brought to light a number of elements that cause accelerated aging. It is interesting to note that the processes that cause early aging of the skin, of the cells in the skin, are the same ones that cause aging in the cells throughout the body. Like the skin, the whole body can age faster or slower...and the whole body can get older without aging. By working out this puzzle made up of hundreds and thousands of studies of aging, we can begin to understand this phenomenon. We can explain what happens within prematurely aging skin and thus in the prematurely aging body. We understand that this process of aging starts in our cells...and that we must take care of our cells!

Why dwell on cells?

The body consists of billions of cells, and each one of them plays a role in the body's proper functioning. Whether in making skin, causing the heart to beat, fighting infection, or locating a memory in the brain, cells are the basis of how the body functions. Cells are living things and the body's health depends on cells being in good condition and healthy.

"...cells are the basis of the proper functioning of tissues and organs, and their maintenance is essential to preventing aging."

A number of differences become apparent in examining aged skin and skin that has not aged or has aged less. Aged skin has lost collagen because, with age, cells make less of it and make it less well. The skin gets dry because the cells of the epidermis are no longer able to build an effective barrier; they are also less effective in making vitamin D. Whether in the skin, blood vessels, or brain, cells are the basis of the proper functioning of tissues and organs, and their maintenance is essential to preventing aging. So let's open the door and enter into this world where we will find a key (*THE KEY?*) to aging. Our objective will be understanding how to gain control over the aging process. In achieving it, we will spend time looking at 5 targets that we can easily act on.

CHAPTER 3

THE KEY: PROTECT AND MAINTAIN THE CELLS THAT STAY WITH US ALL THROUGH LIFE

———

NOTE: This is the most technical chapter. It offers a simple understanding of how the aging process works in the body, but it is not essential for understanding the subsequent chapters, which describe targets and tools.

A quick look at cells and their roles

Our tissues consist of millions of cells, which are the smallest living units of our body. Like little blocks, cells unite to make tissues and organs, such as skin, the heart, and the brain. For tissues and organs to function properly, the cells must remain healthy and live as long as possible. For cells to remain sound and healthy, they must be protected and properly maintained, and their components must remain damaged (Figure 1).

For example:

- The genetic code must remain intact.
- Internal structures (energy production systems, etc.) must function well.
- The cell wall must be made with quality materials (the "good" fats we eat).
- They must be cleaned regularly.

FIGURE 1
The cell and some of its components

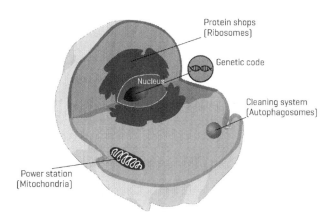

Protein shops
(Ribosomes)

Genetic code

Cleaning system
(Autophagosomes)

Nucleus

Power station
(Mitochondria)

The body's cells have repair systems to maintain their structures. Sometimes, however, the damage is significant or has built up during the life of the cell, making repair impossible. For some cells, those that only live for several days or weeks, a certain amount of damage is of less importance. Other cells, however, have been with us since birth and must remain alive for months or even our whole lives. Damage to these cells results in health consequences in the long run. The appropriate strategy, clearly demonstrated in scientific studies, therefore aims at specifically taking care of the cells that remain with us throughout life.

Thus, the strategy will be simple:

1. *Prevent* **damage to cells and their components.**
2. *Repair and clean* **damaged structures.**
3. *Eliminate cells that are too severely damaged.*

The tools described in this book are intended to activate these processes and act on the body's cells, principally those cells that stay with us throughout life.

Which cells stay with us throughout life?

As seen above, the most important cells to protect and maintain are those that live for a long time, whose proper functioning is essential for maintaining our long-term health. There are mainly two types of cells that remain with us lifelong. First, there are the cells that don't renew themselves, those that are the same since birth. Examples are the neurons in the brain and the cells of the heart. Second, there are *stem cells*: they stay with us throughout life and constantly ensure the production of new cells that serve to renew tissues. That is what happens in the skin, the intestines, and red and white blood cells, tissues that are renewed throughout life from only a few stem cells.

Consider the epidermis (Figure 2): these cells live about 4 weeks before they emerge on the surface and their life ends. Although the cells in our skin are constantly changed, their renewal is the job of only a few cells, at the base of the epidermis, which are the same as at birth. These are the cells called *stem cells*. They must not be damaged. As long as the stem cells and their environment are healthy, production of the epidermis is optimal and it can continue to function well. When the stem cells of the skin are damaged during life, they become fewer and less effective: the epidermis becomes a less solid barrier; healing is slower; hair becomes white or gray.... As a result, the epidermis is more likely to develop problems.

FIGURE 2
The skin, its renewal, its stem cells

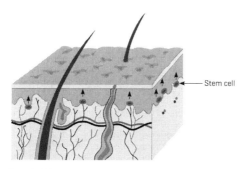

Stem cell

The cells of the epidermis are renewed every 4 weeks. All the cells of the epidermis are produced by only few stem cells. The stem cells has to be preserved because they are with us all through life.

This process—the renewal of tissues by way of a few stem cells—occurs in many other tissues and organs. Keeping stem cells in good condition is therefore an essential objective for maintaining the body in good working order, because damage to these cells ultimately affects tissues and organs. For example, accumulated damage to muscle stem cells causes a loss in muscle mass and less effective repair. Damage to the stem cells of white blood cells, which are produced in the bone marrow, makes the immune system less effective. Over the years, the accumulated damage to stem cells winds up negatively affecting our overall health.

As mentioned earlier, in addition to stem cells, the other cells to be protected are those that don't renew themselves and remain for a very long time or even a whole lifetime, such as heart and brain cells. The brain, which holds our memories, emotions, and personality, is itself susceptible to cellular damage. Preserving this type of cell will therefore also be one of our objectives. The following chapters provide a closer look at what causes damage to cells and what can be done to avoid such damage.

So, whether stem cells responsible for renewing tissue (skin, intestines, etc.) and organs (liver, adrenal glands, etc.) or cells that last throughout a lifetime (heart, brain, etc.), they must be kept alive and in good condition if the body is to continue to function effectively over a long period. Allowing damage to accumulate opens the door to aging, degenerative diseases, and cancer. Let's see how.

What happens to cells when they are damaged?

We have seen that the cells that accompany us throughout life must be properly cared for. To understand aging, we must understand what happens to these cells when they are damaged. First, damage can occur in various cell structures, such as the genetic code, energy-production systems, and cell envelope. Once damaged, cells may be repaired by their own repair system. Sometimes, however, the damage the cell has experienced over time is such that it can no longer be restored to a normal state.

So, what becomes of cells that, over the years, have undergone irreparable damage? This is an important question, and its answer IS THE KEY CONCEPT in understanding the aging process and the appearance of age-related diseases. The body generally has two main options when a cell experiences irreparable damage (Figure 3):

1. *Not intervene* and allow the cell to try to perform its role, even though it has not been 100% repaired.
2. *Allow the cell to enter senescence.* That's a new word. Roughly, it means sidelining the cell, preventing it from dividing to prevent it from continuing to damage itself.

In the following section, we will see that neither of these scenarios is helpful for our body. Allowing cells to drift toward one of these two scenarios is the start of the WHOLE process of aging, degenerative disease, and a fertile ground for cancer. It is most likely the cause of our spending the last 10 to 15 years of life in poorer health (the difference between life expectancy and health expectancy). WE MUST THEREFORE INTERVENE FIRST, so that our cells don't have to make this choice.

What happens to the body when its cells are pushed toward the abyss of senescence?

We have just seen that when cells have experienced irreparable damage, the body must make a choice that will have consequences on our health. Let's look at the impact of the two principal options stem cells have when they are damaged (Figure 3). This will allow us to understand why aging, cancer, and degenerative disease are related.

The *first option* is for the body to allow the stem cells to continue to function despite the damage. Remember that stem cells are responsible for making tissues and organs (e.g., skin, intestine, and lungs). The cell may therefore continue to do its work (for example, producing epidermis) but remains more vulnerable than a healthy cell. The consequence of this choice is an increased risk of transforming the damaged cell into a cancerous one. This path thus opens the door to cancers.

The *second option* is for the body to sideline the cell, allowing it to become senescent. Senescence is one of the most powerful protection mechanisms the body has against cancer. Cellular senescence means that the cell stops renewing itself, thus protecting itself from imminent death or being transformed into a cancer cell. This, however, results in a loss of valuable stem cells, which are essential for making new tissue (for example, skin) and organs (for example, muscles, the immune system). This process is also generally irreversible, and not without consequences. The first consequence is that the loss of these stem cells results in organs and tissues being imperfectly regenerated and becoming less effective in performing their functions. In other words, the tissues age. The second consequence is that, in addition to reducing organ efficacy, this powerful protection against cancer increases inflammation in tissues and promotes degenerative diseases (osteoarthritis, atherosclerosis, macular degeneration, chronic respiratory diseases). As the body ages, the number of its cells undergoing senescence increases. This produces even more inflammation and makes the situation worse. So, it is better for the body not to reach the point of having to create senescent cells. Over the years, the burden of accumulated senescent cells in tissues continues to rise. It is therefore necessary to promote the elimination of these senescent cells by a process that might be called "senolysis." (We will revisit this later).

FIGURE 3
The key: the fate of damaged cells

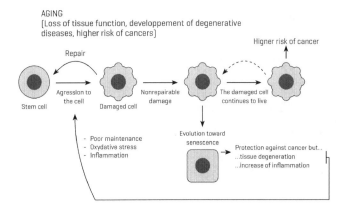

AGING
[Loss of tissue function, developpement of degenerative diseases, higher risk of cancers]

To illustrate this process, let's take the example of what happens in the skin (Figure 4). As a person ages, the number of senescent cells in both the dermis and epidermis increases, while there are fewer and fewer healthy stem cells. On the one hand, a reduction of stem cells makes tissue production less efficient. On the other, the presence of even only a few senescent cells attracts white blood cells, which provokes tissue inflammation. This contributes to destroying collagen and causes even more damage to neighboring cells. Consequently, the skin takes on a more wrinkled appearance and becomes more fragile; its pigmentation becomes irregular, it makes less vitamin D, and precancerous cells appear.

Impact on the skin of the accumulation of damaged cells

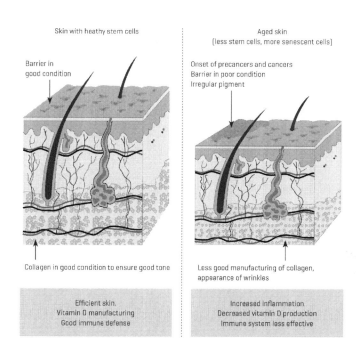

Skin with heathy stem cells

Aged skin
[less stem cells, more senescent cells]

Barrier in
good condition

Onset of precancers and cancers
Barrier in poor condition
Irregular pigment

Collagen in good condition to ensure good tone

Less good manufacturing of collagen,
appearance of wrinkles

Efficient skin.
Vitamin D manufacturing
Good immune defense

Increased inflammation
Decreased vitamin D production
Immune system less effective

It is not just the skin that is affected: the whole body falls victim to cell senescence. Senses (taste, smell, hearing) become less effective; the same applies to the cartilage in joints, to muscles, and to the whole body.

In the light of today's knowledge, the key to aging seems to lie in this concept. It would explain how aging, degenerative diseases, and cancer result from the same process. The body must decide every day what it will do with the cells that are starting to be damaged and are no longer capable of being repaired. If it doesn't intervene but allows these cells continue to function, cancerous tumors can develop. To protect us from cancer, the body can also stop the cells from doing their jobs (activate senescence), which reduces the quantity of stem cells and, accordingly, decreases the quality and effectiveness of tissues and organs. In other words, they age. The presence of senescent cells in the tissues promotes local inflammation, thereby exposing us to degenerative diseases.

"In the light of today's knowledge, the key to aging seems to lie in this concept."

Since these three elements (accelerated aging, cancers, degenerative diseases) increase with age and result from the same process, we ought to do something to prevent our cells from entering the abyss of senescence, that "key" to aging. This new understanding of how cells function makes it possible for us to define a strategy to ward off these age-related conditions. This strategy seeks to prevent damage as well as to repair and clean cells. To this purpose, we will examine the 5 most relevant targets in the following chapters. Reaching these targets will require the use of concrete, effective, and easily adoptable tools to protect and properly maintain our cells.

But before looking at our intervention strategies, keep in mind that not all the processes leading to aging produce symptoms. Therefore, we need to act with conviction and remember that physiological studies support our actions and our work in achieving these goals.

CHAPTER 4

TARGET 1: OXIDATION

DO YOUR OWN "ANTI-RUST" TREATMENTS

What is oxidation and oxidative stress?

As you make your way down supermarket aisles, you can see shelves stocked with antioxidant supplements, antioxidant cookies, and even antioxidant soft drinks. Antioxidants seem to be what many supplement and food manufacturers want us to take to prevent all sorts of health problems. But what is oxidation, what is oxidative stress, and do we need antioxidant supplements?

Oxidation is a little like rust. On a car, rust caused by oxygen can affect a number of parts. Small rust spots may appear here and there without much in the way of consequences initially. But if no anti-rust treatment is applied, the process spreads, weakening the whole structure.

The situation is not so straightforward in our cells. The oxidation reactions caused by oxygen are important and even essential for cells to work properly and for immune-system functioning. Since the body needs oxidation, it must not be completely blocked, as that could be harmful to the body. When oxidation reactions get to a certain level in a cell, its natural antioxidant systems are overwhelmed, leading to a situation called *oxidative stress*, when too much oxidation occurs. In the presence of oxidative stress, damage starts to occur in the cells, and all the structures (cell wall, genetic code, etc.) can be affected. The damage can become irreparable, with the consequences described above. (Figure 5).

FIGURE 5
Impact of oxidative stress

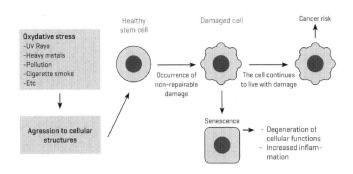

How does oxidative stress impact health?

We have seen that excess oxidation and oxidative stress damage cells. If the damage becomes irreparable, the cells are pushed to the edge of the abyss. As explained in the preceding chapter, such cells risk becoming cancerous; they are also at greater risk of becoming senescent and causing the body to age prematurely.

The premature aging caused by excess oxidation contributes to conditions associated with premature aging:

- various cancers
- atherosclerosis
- aging of the skin (pigment irregularities, wrinkles)
- macular degeneration
- presbycusis (hearing loss)
- chronic bronchitis
- dementias and Alzheimer's disease
- erectile dysfunction
- Parkinson's disease
- cataracts

What causes excess oxidation?

We have seen that the oxidant–antioxidant balance is important for cells to work properly and that problems begin when excessive oxidation occurs. Let's look at some factors that can lead to excessive oxidation.

First of all, one of the greatest producers of oxidative stress—ultraviolet radiation—has special significance for the skin and eyes. It damages skin cells, causes the skin to age more quickly, and increases the risk of cancer. As for the eyes, it increases the risk of cataracts and macular degeneration. One of the other causes that must not be overlooked is smoking, which generates major oxidative stress in the lungs and throughout the body.

While ultraviolet radiation and smoking can easily be avoided, other causes are much harder to steer clear of. Among the most insidious causes of oxidative stress are atmospheric pollution, heavy metals, certain types of radiation, excess calories and sugar, and even psychological stress! Since all the sources of excess oxidation cannot be avoided, adopting protective habits that counteract oxidative stress would seem justified.

Tools protecting against oxidative stress
Tool 1. The paradox of physical exercise

Much has been said about the benefits of physical activity, so I will just point out a few essential elements drawn from the scientific literature. It has been clearly demonstrated that physical activity increases life expectancy. First, changing from a sedentary lifestyle to a more physically active one (such as brisk walking for half an hour, 5 times a week) will add about 3 years a person's lifespan, which is a good start. In recent years, researchers have also discovered that muscle contraction releases substances that are beneficial for the whole body. Exercise can stimulate the immune system, improve cognitive functions, and even keep the skin looking more youthful! It has also been demonstrated that physical effort (muscle exertion with increased heart rate and respiration) and maintaining physical fitness allow muscles to produce even more of these substances. You can extend your lifespan by up to 7 years by engaging in regular physical exercise.

The effect of physical activity on oxidative stress contributes, in part, to its health benefits. First, paradoxically, physical activity generates oxidation that then stimulates numerous antioxidative mechanisms. Second, the contraction of muscles promotes the release of a number of substances throughout the body, some of which reduce oxidative stress. Physical activity therefore acts as a powerful activator of antioxidative (and also anti-inflammatory) systems and remains one of the best ways of counteracting oxidation.

Tool 2. Sleep well...

Sliding between the sheets of a comfortable bed, spending the nights in the arms of Morpheus, dreaming beautiful dreams and getting up the next morning, fresh, and ready to tackle the day... Many dream of just that. A good night's sleep lets you feel more energetic. And people who sleep better are perceived as being healthier and more attractive. All good reasons for wanting a good night's sleep!

In addition to leaving a person feeling tired, poorer sleep is associated with a higher risk of developing various health problems. Sleeping poorly has negative effects on the mechanisms associated with aging: increased oxidative stress and blood markers of subclinical inflammation (discussed in the next chapter). Moreover, a study of men in their sixties has shown that just one night of disturbed sleep causes an increase in cellular senescence (as mentioned above, the accumulation of senescent cells is a marker of tissue aging). Bad nights thus slowly eat away at health. Conversely, sound sleep helps fight oxidative stress in the body and brain. It also helps to literally remove certain toxic substances from brain cells. It therefore seems important to take up habits that promote sleep. Here are some that have demonstrated their benefits in various studies.

Some tips for a better night's sleep

- Get exposure to light early and keep the room well-lit during the day.
- Have a breakfast that is high in tryptophan, an amino acid abundant in a variety of foods such as legumes, nuts, and eggs.
- Engage in physical activity.
- Avoid stimulants.
- Lower ambient lighting about 90 minutes before bedtime.
- Select your bedtime based on when you want to get up and the desired amount of sleep. For example, if you want to get up at 6 a.m. and you sleep 7 hours on average, set your bedtime at around 11 p.m.
- The bedroom should be as dark as possible and cool.
- Treat sleep apnea and various discomforts (pain, itching, etc.)
- Relax and forget your worries for a while (write them down...and sleep on it!)
- Certain foods, infusions, and supplements have been proven to promote more restful sleep (valerian, hops, lemon balm, passiflora, cherries, kiwis, salmon, magnesium).

Tool 3. Put "anti-rusting" foods in your shopping cart

Look no further. The variety of vegetables you put in

your grocery cart will do the job. In fact, a supplement could never provide such a wide variety of antioxidants. For example, eating just 1 or 2 Brazil nuts is sufficient to activate certain antioxidant systems. Numerous fruits, vegetables, nuts, and herbs have shown similar benefits. Just imagine if you combined several of them! What you put in your grocery cart should be selected to activate this anti-aging system and deliver many other health benefits.

So...

As mentioned at the start of this chapter, the oxidant–antioxidant system is a complex chain of reactions that is very important for the body's balance. Excess oxidation causes oxidative stress and contributes to accelerated aging. But, in the light of certain studies, breaking one link in this chain with a high dose of an antioxidant supplement could also be harmful to health. For example, one study has even shown that high doses of beta-carotene (which has known antioxidant action) could increase the risk of lung cancer in smokers. And this is not the only study reaching similar conclusions. So, a smarter approach would a more general one, as described above.

In fact, the things that facilitate good sleep promote higher secretion of melatonin, which is an important antioxidant for the brain. Physical activity is a powerful stimulant of antioxidant systems, and eating a variety of vegetables promotes a more overall activation of the body's protective systems. This economical and balanced approach is therefore preferable to supplements for optimizing body functioning in order to achieve healthy longevity.

CHAPTER 5

TARGET 2: INFLAMMATION

PUT OUT THE FIRES

———

What is inflammation and what is its impact?

Let's take the example of a bacterium that causes a skin infection. The skin swells, reddens, and becomes sensitive: this is inflammation rising to the body's defense and hunting down the invaders. Inflammation is useful to all mammals: it plays a role in survival by participating in the fight against infections. It is also involved in healing wounds and many other functions. Once its job has been done, however, the inflammation process should turn off and shut down.

Sometimes the inflammatory process is activated without our knowing it. This is referred to as subclinical inflammation, which is another way of saying that we don't feel it, but it can still be detected in blood tests. This low-level inflammation keeps the body in a state of combat, causing an accumulation of damage to tissues and cells over the years (Figure 6). This unnecessary fight, which goes on without our knowing it, attracts white cells to tissues (skin, joints, brain, etc.). Accordingly, the body must make new white cells at an accelerated pace and that, over time, can exhaust the immune system, making it less effective. This whole process favors premature aging of the body and the immune system, and results (over the long term) in numerous health consequences.

"This low-level inflammation keeps the body in a state of combat, causing an accumulation of damage to tissues and cells."

FIGURE 6
Long-term impact of inflammation

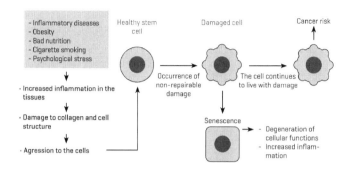

What are the health consequences of chronic inflammation?

Such low-level inflammation, experienced over years (also called chronic inflammation) can damage cells, destroy collagen, and make all tissues more fragile. In the skin, it can promote accelerated aging and the development of cancers, both on the portions exposed to the sun and those unexposed. For the body, in addition to contributing to premature aging, it is involved in the development of a number of degenerative conditions and diseases:

- Atherosclerosis
- Cardiovascular diseases
- Erectile dysfunction
- Dementias and Alzheimer's disease

- Parkinson's disease
- Accelerated aging of the skin (collagen destruction)
- Sarcopenia and frailty in the elderly
- Arthritis
- Osteoporosis
- Macular degeneration
- Hearing loss
- Fatigue

In addition to damaging certain tissues, this underlying inflammation modifies how the brain functions. Some researchers have seen a link between increased signs of inflammation in the blood and declining psychomotor performance and memory. Chronic inflammation may even reduce testosterone in men (and testosterone contributes to reducing inflammation!), provoke a sense of fatigue, make the body more sensitive to pain, and promote depression (see sidebar). With all these consequences, not only for the aging of organs and various age-related diseases, but also for quality of life, it is important to identify the causes of inflammation and how to counteract them.

"Some researchers have seen a link between increased signs of inflammation in the blood and declining psychomotor performance and memory."

Why does inflammation, even when just subclinical, make us feel depressed?

We have seen that the mechanisms that lead to accelerated aging do not cause symptoms, yet there is at least one exception with respect to the link between depression and inflammation. To understand the origin of these symptoms, we must look to mammalian history. First, it is important to know that, as mammals and human beings have evolved, the main cause of inflammation has always been infection, because the inflammatory reaction is essential to fighting infection. When we get a cold or the flu, we feel unwell and a little depressed, along with having a cough, runny nose, and sore throat. Feeling depressed during an infection forces us to limit our outdoor activities, allowing us to preserve our energy for fighting infection. Moreover, a depressed mood favors social isolation, which prevents contamination of others. So, the depressive state generated by inflammation would have been a survival factor for individuals and species for thousands of years. Moreover, researchers have discovered a mechanism in the brain that fosters a depressive state when inflammation occurs. Nowadays, we can treat infections better, but the various sources of inflammation (such as obesity and psoriasis, for example), even if they are not infectious in origin, are also factors promoting these same depressive symptoms. Understanding this phenomenon gives us an additional reason to intervene to reduce the inflammation that is surreptitiously raging in our bodies.

What causes subclinical inflammation?

Don't let inflammatory diseases go untreated

While a number of types of inflammatory diseases affect one or another part of the body, some do more to increase general inflammation in the body as a whole. For example, an inflammation of the skin (such as psoriasis), in the joints (such as rheumatoid arthritis), or even in the mouth (gingivitis) leaves traces in the blood. It is important to note that subclinical inflammation is not the source of these diseases: they generate the inflammation. Even if the inflammation is located in just one organ or one type of tissue, blood tests can serve to measure the inflammation and to show that the whole body is affected by its consequences.

Effective treatment of these diseases therefore not only helps reduce their symptoms, but also diminishes the signs of inflammation in the blood, as well as the harmful consequences referred to in the preceding paragraph. Thus, anyone with a chronic inflammatory disease has every reason to seek out effective treatment. Unfortunately, infections and inflammatory diseases are not the only sources of inflammation: researchers have found signs of inflammation in the blood in other contexts, some of which are surprising, as we will see.

Obesity: a cause of manageable inflammation.

The evidence is growing that a high body-mass index fosters a number of health problems. The accumulation of fat, both on the body surface and in tissues like muscles and the liver, causes a number of changes in the body and promotes effects that include chronic inflammation throughout the body. This chronic inflammation could represent the link between obesity and a number of health problems. And to complicate the situation, this small subclinical inflammation seems to contribute to the development of obesity. Conversely, it has been clearly demonstrated that weight loss reduces blood-inflammation rates. Achieving and maintaining a healthy weight therefore is an essential objective for keeping the risks of degenerative diseases as low as possible and thereby limiting premature aging.

"It has been clearly demonstrated that weight loss lowers blood-inflammation rates."

Other insidious causes of subclinical inflammation

In recent years, more sensitive laboratory tests have made

it possible to identify other causes of inflammation that disrupt the body's functioning. Among the other factors causing increased inflammation in blood and body tissues are smoking, a diet too high in sugar or saturated fats, lack of sleep, and psychological stress. In fact, it has been demonstrated that people who were mistreated as children tend to maintain a higher inflammatory state as adults. Finally, the level of inflammation in the body tends to rise gradually with age.

So let's examine a few simple measures that could help offset this insidious phenomenon. They contribute not only to slowing down the illnesses associated with it, but could also, as we have seen, have a real impact on psychological well-being.

Tools for fighting subclinical inflammation
Tool 4: Target and maintain a healthy weight.

As mentioned above, the accumulation of fat generates inflammation throughout the body. Correcting overweight is thus an important objective for limiting the body's needless aging. While having a specialist's advice can be a major asset in this regard, some simple and sometimes surprising measures (backed by evidence) can be applied immediately.

Some tips to help maintain a healthy weight

- Make physical activity a part of your daily routine.
- Avoid a sedentary lifestyle (different from "engaging in physical activity").
- Comply with the recommended calorie intake.
- Cut out all sweetened drinks.
- Prefer solid foods because chewing helps suppress appetite.
- Eat a high-protein breakfast.
- Eat a high-fiber diet.
- Add herbs and spices to help feel satiated.
- Avoid late snacks (at night).
- Be sure to sleep well.
- Get good exposure to light, starting in the morning.
- Use smaller plates.
- Maintain good intestinal flora.

Tool 5. Dark fruits and vegetables

The many pigments that plants display make walks in nature more pleasant and send signals to many insects and animals. One of these pigments, called anthocyanin, has been the subject of numerous health studies. Anthocyanins give fruits and vegetables colors ranging from red to purple to blue. Both animal and human studies have shown that this pigment family has anti-inflammatory effects. But even more interesting are two studies of a group of nearly 2,000 women ranging in age from 18 to 76 years, which clearly demonstrated that consuming vegetables containing anthocyanins—fruits and vegetables with lots of red, blue, or purple—was associated with reduced signs of inflammation in the blood. The following table gives a list of foods high in anthocyanins...and there's plenty to choose from. Moreover, tea, coffee, cocoa, garlic, turmeric, and ginger also provide anti-inflammatory benefits. As you can see, there are a lot of good choices!

Foods high in anthocyanins

Acai berries, black beans, black plums, blackberries, blackcurrants, blood oranges, blue corn, blueberries, cherries, chokeberries, cranberries, elderberries, raspberries, red cabbage, red grapes, and strawberries

Tool 6. Cultivate the right bacteria

Intestinal flora, cutaneous flora, and *microbiome* are all terms that are slowly becoming part of our vocabulary for describing the bacteria living on our bodies. We are only beginning to discover the beneficial (or harmful) impact of certain types of bacteria present on our bodies (in the skin, mouth, digestive system). Intestinal flora (especially in the large intestine) have been studied most, but, even there, we are just seeing the tip of the iceberg. Our intestinal flora consists of billions of bacteria that interact with our digestive and immune systems, as well as other parts of the body, and can really affect how they function. A varied flora not only makes it possible to better withstand the intestinal changes induced by antibiotics, but could also have a beneficial effect in controlling obesity, on the immune system and the brain, and on the risks of allergy, asthma, and eczema.

The benefits are therefore felt all the way to the surface: because of its effect on inflammation, a healthy intestinal flora can even contribute to maintaining healthy skin. Some probiotics (e.g., *Lactobacillus johnsonii*) help make the skin more tolerant of the sun. Others (e.g. *Lactobacillus rueteri*) reduce skin inflammation in mice and give their skin a younger appearance.

"...because of its effect on inflammation, a healthy intestinal flora can even contribute to maintaining healthy skin."

As for subclinical inflammation, the beneficial effect of good intestinal flora is undeniable. It has even been demonstrated that the influence of intestinal flora on inflammation begins at the age of 2, and probably long before. Certain strains of probiotics in particular have an anti-inflammatory effect (e.g. *Bifidobacterium breve, Lactobacillus casei, Lactobacillus helveticus, Lactobacillus rhamnosus,* and *Lactobacillus salivarius*). Probiotics are only a part of the equation, because bacterial supplements have just a temporary effect on inflammation. Still, maintaining good intestinal flora is vital for the long term. Ever heard of prebiotics?

To maintain good flora, the "good" bacteria have to be nourished with what are called prebiotics. For example, a diet high in soluble fibers (garlic, onions, whole-grain cereals, legumes, nuts, and bananas), whole grains, and polyphenols (found in numerous plants) contributes to promoting the growth of good bacteria. Moreover, habits like physical activity and maintaining a healthy weight help establish a richer flora that is healthier for the body. On the other hand, smoking; a sedentary lifestyle; irregular sleep patterns; and the consumption of saturated fats, antibiotics, or certain drugs to control gastric acidity can all have a harmful effect on intestinal flora and thus how the entire body functions.

We cannot live without these bacteria in our body; they contribute to digestion, make vitamins, defend us against infections, and lots more. These bacteria have a vested interest in us living a long time...and, to help us be healthy, we really should maintain good bacterial flora. It's a win–win situation!

Tool 7. Just a simple tip in passing!

Even if we don't dwell on the subject, you should know that the links between psychological stress and the processes that lead to premature aging have been well established, and that there are several possible approaches to reducing such stress. Sometimes seeing a psychologist can help in working through problems; sometimes pursuits like meditation or "full consciousness" can help better manage psychological stress and improve well-being. But, surprisingly enough, one very simple tool—the way we breathe—not only can offset the reactions that psychological stress creates in the body but also reduces subclinical inflammation, thereby lessening the oxidative stress in cells! Diaphragmatic (or abdominal) breathing at a rate of about 6 breaths per minute for 15 minutes, activates the parasympathetic nervous system, with a calming effect that contributes to reducing the body's stress reflexes. Activation of this system succeeds in slowing inflammation in various ways, including a direct action on certain white blood cells, and it has an antioxidant effect on certain organs. Simple and effective!

"...one very simple tool—the way we breathe—not only can offset the reactions that psychological stress creates in the body but also reduces subclinical inflammation..."

Tool 8. Omega-3 fatty acids: the finishing touch

Omega-3 fatty acid supplements often take up a lot of space on the food-supplement shelves. Their labels boast "helps cardiovascular health" and "boosts brain functioning." In fact, the literature brings out many other benefits. Omega-3 fatty acids, especially those from marine sources, (eicosapentaenoic acid or EPA and docosahexaenoic acid or DHA) have a number of actions. One of their important contributions to health is their effect on inflammation. Generally, consuming omega-3 fatty acids not only promotes a reduction in inflammation but, in addition, it *resolves* the inflammatory process. Medicine now understands that inflammation does not subside on its own, but is reduced by an active resolution process that involves the presence of omega-3 fatty acids in cells. It also seems that this inflammation resolution process tends to function less well with age. We therefore obtain numerous benefits from including dietary fish (about 2 portions per week) or a good supplement of omega-3 fatty acids (several times a week) to help in resolving inflammation.

So...

Subclinical inflammation is increasingly recognized as a driver of aging. A number of scientific articles already use a term to designate this phenomenon: *inflammaging*. This process can be offset by certain simple actions. So don't let inflammation consume your body and depress your days...put out the fires!

CHAPTER 6

TARGET 3: GLYCATION

DON'T LET YOUR GOOSE BE COOKED!

———

What is glycation?

When you grill a piece of meat until it is nicely browned, it takes on that flavor that will delight your guests. The heat causes the sugars and proteins contained in the meat to react, the taste to change, and the texture to become more tender because bonds are created within the meat by proteins binding to sugars. This reaction, which connects and binds the various parts of the piece of meat is called *glycation* and leads to the creation of glycation end products. This same reaction can also occur inside the body, where it generates functional problems and is responsible for the *needless aging* of the body's cells.

But don't worry, your goose isn't cooked! There are solutions! Let's begin by taking a first look at how glycation occurs in the body and explain how it can be halted. We will also see the impact of consuming foods that contain glycation end products and provide a few simple tips on how to reduce their impact.

How does glycation take place in the body?

Unlike what happens when a piece of meat is being cooked, the glycation process (which ultimately binds the proteins to sugars in our cells and tissues) occurs rather slowly in the body over a few weeks to a few months. The blood-glucose level drives the formation of these toxic products. If the blood-sugar level rises substantially on occasion or is often high, glycation progresses more quickly. Take the example of what goes on in red blood cells. Doctors can measure the level of glycated hemoglobin (the amount of hemoglobin that has undergone glycation from the rise in the blood-sugar level) in the blood of diabetics. The more often the blood-sugar level has been high, and especially if it has been substantially high, the more the hemoglobin becomes glycated. On the other hand, after the blood-sugar level has been adequately controlled for a number of weeks, the new red blood cells will be less glycated and return to normal. Although glycation in the body is higher in people whose blood-sugar levels are poorly controlled (like diabetics), even non-diabetics can fall victim to it. As discussed below, this highlights the importance of all of us reducing the consumption of foods that cause blood-sugar levels to rise.

It's not just red blood cells that can become glycated: all cells in the body—including collagen and even nails—can be affected. When blood-sugar levels remain low, the new cells and the new collagen (some collagen fibers may take up to 10 to 15 years to be renewed!) will not be affected by this condition. This is actually good news: we can reduce the glycation end products in our bodies. Now let's turn to glycation's tangible consequences.

What is the impact of glycation in the body?

All body tissues can be affected by glycation. Let's first look at what happens in the skin (Figure 7). The entire epidermis and dermis can undergo glycation, but skin exposed to the sun, the skin of diabetics, and the skin of smokers are more seriously affected. The bonding of sugars and proteins causes the skin loses its elasticity. Its level of inflammation goes up, and the skin's and body's natural antioxidants become less effective. The skin heals more slowly and becomes more vulnerable to sun damage. Glycation can result in accelerated cell senescence, both in the dermis and epidermis. The increases in the body's blood-sugar level, which would appear rather innocuous, actually cause many functional problems in the body's tissues. And not only the skin is affected by glycation: the changes described above can also be observed in other organs. The following are some examples of how glycation affects health.

FIGURE 7
Impact of glycation

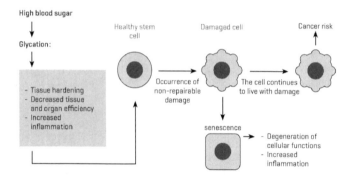

In the rest of the body, glycation can contribute to:

· hardening of blood vessels;
· causing cataracts and macular degeneration;
· disrupting the functioning of the female reproductive system;
· reducing muscular strength and physical performance;
· increasing the risk of bone fractures;

- making the cartilage and disks between vertebras more fragile;
- reducing kidney filtration; and
- disrupting antioxidizing and cell cleaning systems. (Cleaning systems will be revisited in in Chapter 8.)

What is the impact of glycation end products from outside the body?

We have just seen that the glycation occurring in the body has harmful effects on health, but what about glycation that occurs outside the body that is ingested or inhaled? Some foods contain high levels of glycation end products: this is especially true of sausage, meats, and fats that have been grilled, roasted, or fried. Raw, boiled, stewed, and steamed foods contain relatively little. Incidentally, cigarette smoke contains a lot of these end products.

When these substances are ingested or inhaled, a portion is absorbed into the blood and their toxic effects are felt throughout the body. Overall, their main impact is to increase inflammation and oxidative stress in tissues... our top two targets! On the other hand, studies show that reducing the intake of foods high in glycation end products (grilled meats, sausage) decreases the blood inflammation markers that show up in laboratory tests. The impact is real and measurable.

Tools protecting against glycation

Tool +. Golden rule: avoid causing blood-sugar levels to rise

Since increased blood-sugar level is the main factor promoting glycation in the body, avoiding higher blood-sugar levels must be an objective. Of course, proper control of blood-sugar levels is vital in diabetics. But even people who are not diabetic should limit their intake of sweetened drinks or products containing refined sugars like glucose and fructose as much as possible. It has also been clearly demonstrated that opting for whole foods and integrating fiber and legumes in the diet help control blood sugar. Yet a selective diet is not the only way to go. Avoiding a sedentary lifestyle is also beneficial. A brisk walk 15 minutes after a meal or even a 2-minute walk every 20 minutes helps keep blood-sugar levels in check. These habits reap real benefits for the body. For example, adopting good eating habits can reduce the amount of glycated collagen by 25% in just 4 months. While controlling blood sugar is the basic strategy for reducing the formation of glycation products, other ingredients can also contribute.

Tool 9. Vinegar to the rescue

Vinegar can play a number of roles in the kitchen, but science has discovered that vinegar has at least two health benefits. First, adding vinegar (or lemon juice) to foods before cooking them reduces the formation of glycation products. Remember that food glycation promotes inflammation in the body. Marinades are therefore not only tasty, but have a real impact on health. In addition, studies have shown that vinegar can reduce rises in blood-sugar levels and insulin in humans, whether they are diabetic or not. Just a little vinegar (10 mL or 2 teaspoons)—even just in salad dressing—seems to have benefits on the higher blood-sugar levels that occur after eating.

Tool 10. Get spices and herbs out of the cupboard

Some spices and herbs have antioxidant effects, while others have anti-inflammatory effects. Many studies have also shown that they are effective in fighting glycation reactions (see the table). Adding spices to food before cooking it offers additional benefits and reduces the formation of certain toxic products. A study compared hamburger patties seasoned with a mixture of herbs and spices to unseasoned ones. After cooking, the seasoned patties contained fewer products toxic to the genetic code and fewer products promoting glycation in the body. Thus, foods seasoned with herbs and spices before cooking really caused less damage to the body. That makes another reason for seasoning food, in addition to pleasing the palate. Yet not only herbs and spices offer these benefits: other plants are anti-glycation agents, including fresh and aged garlic, onions, hibiscus, and green tea.

Herbs and spices that demonstrate anti-glycation effects
- Allspice
- Basil
- Cinnamon
- Cloves
- Coriander seeds
- Cumin
- Ginger
- Marjoram
- Oregano
- Parsley
- Pepper
- Rosemary
- Sage
- Tarragon
- Thyme
- Turmeric

So...

Glycation disrupts the body's functioning and increases the effectiveness of processes that promote premature aging (oxidative stress, inflammation). The good news is that we can "lose" glycation end products over months and years. Adopting certain habits described above will stop glycation in the body's organs, enabling them to resume optimal functioning. Really, your goose is not cooked!

CHAPTER 7

TARGET 4: TELOMERES

AVOID WEAR AND TEAR ON YOUR GENETIC CODE

———

What are telomeres?

Think of a pair of your running shoes and imagine that every time you put them on, you cut a little bit off each end of your shoelaces. They get shorter and shorter and start to unravel until you can no longer tie them. At that point, the shoes are no longer safe to wear; you would be better off leaving them in the closet. Well, the same is true for cells!

As we know, each cell contains chromosomes that hold the individual's genetic code. Telomeres are the tips of chromosomes, a little like the ends of a shoelace (Figure

8). They contribute to keeping the genetic code stable and are important in reducing the risk of cells becoming cancerous. Each time that a cell renews itself, a bit of the telomeres—and therefore a tiny bit of genetic code—is cut off. The telomeres become shorter each time a cell regenerates or divides. When the telomeres are too short, after a certain number of renewals (several years), the cell stops multiplying and enters a senescence process. It is sidelined, which provides, as noted above, some protection against cancer. But this protection against cancer comes at a price, because an accumulation of senescent cells is a major element in the development of age-related diseases and the body's aging. Telomere erosion therefore affects health.

FIGURE 8
Consequences of short telomeres on cells

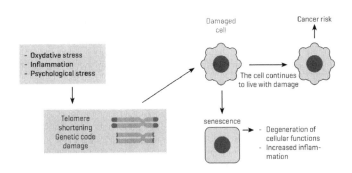

What are the links between telomeres and health?

Generally speaking, telomere length seems to reflect the aging of the body. For example, when elderly men are compared to elderly women, the women, on average, have longer telomeres. Moreover, women generally have a longer life expectancy than men. Some studies seem to associate potential health expectancy with telomere length: longer telomeres equate to longer good health. Other studies seem to show longer telomeres are linked to longer maintenance of cognitive functions.

Conversely, people with shorter telomeres have a greater risk of developing cancer, having a heart attack, contracting a cold, dying of infection, or dying prematurely. People with chronic diseases (cardiovascular diseases, insulin resistance, dementia, chronic obstructive pulmonary disease) generally have shorter telomeres. So, there are many good reasons for examining what influences telomere length.

What promotes short telomeres?

First of all, as we should expect, oxidative stress and inflammation promote accelerated telomere erosion. For example, chronic inflammation, which requires an increase in white-blood-cell production, forces the immune system's stem cells to renew themselves more often. That, in turn, results in accelerated shortening of the telomeres and premature aging of the immune system. Other factors related to telomere shortening cited in the medical literature include smoking, obesity and, in the case of skin cells, ultraviolet rays. Other studies show that areas of skin exposed to the sun have shorter telomeres than unexposed skin. As regards diet, people who consume lots of sweetened drinks or sausages also have shorter telomeres. These are the very same factors identified in the sections herein on oxidative stress and inflammation.

"Intrauterine life and infancy are therefore major determinants of telomere length, and this impact is felt throughout a person's life"

It is interesting to note that studies show that people who have experienced psychological stress, chronic depression, or extended anxiety as well as those who are hostile or pessimistic have shorter telomeres: this can result in up to ten years of accelerated aging! Mothers of gravely ill children may have telomere aging markers that are 9 to 17 years more advanced than otherwise. In addition, individuals exposed to stress during intrauterine life have shorter telomeres when they reach young adulthood. Intrauterine life and childhood are therefore major determinants of telomere length, and this impact is felt throughout a person's life. Given all these elements that wear down telomeres, will we be powerless victims of what we experienced as children for the rest of our lives?

Can telomeres be lengthened?

That is a question that many scientists have tried to answer...and with good reason! We have seen that, when telomeres become too short (after a given number of cellular renewals or as the result of damage to the genetic code), the cell becomes senescent and stops renewing itself. So why do cancer cells endlessly renew themselves? Do they have a special secret? Comparing the cells of certain cancers to noncancerous cells and skin-cancer cells to healthy skin cells, for example, reveals that cancerous cells often use a telomere extension system or telomerase. Telomerase is a enzyme in cells that allows bits of DNA to be added (extending the "shoelaces") to slow down telomere shortening. By maintaining telomere length, cell senescence or death is avoided or postponed. A number of other types of cancer act similarly. But what about healthy, noncancerous cells? Can they benefit from telomerase?

The old notion that telomeres only shorten has now been confronted with new studies. They show that shortening can be slowed (and even, possibly, that telomeres can be lengthened) by activating telomerase in stem cells, which allows cells to enjoy a longer life. But does telomerase activity have a real and measurable impact on health? It seems that it does! Some recent small studies show that good telomerase activity seems to be associated with a lower risk of developing certain cancers and protects our neurons from the damage of oxidative stress. As for the skin, telomerase is more active in the epidermis and dermis of nonsmokers than in the skin of smokers (it has long been known that smoking is a factor that promotes premature aging of the skin). Another study shows that telomerase reactivation allows aged skin to recover and behave like younger skin without increasing the risk of cancer. So, although studies on telomerase are relatively new, a beneficial link along these lines appears to be taking shape.

Tools +. Tools to activate telomerase

So, here are some tools that, according to certain small studies, could stimulate telomerase. These include meditation, physical exercise, a diet high in vegetables, derivatives of certain plants (e.g., extracts of gingko biloba, astragalus, and turmeric root), calorie restriction (this will be revisited), and resveratrol (a polyphenol present in certain plants, among other sources; see resveratrol in the next chapter.)

So...

Although we are not born equal and do not reach adulthood as equals with respect to telomere length, telomere maintenance seems to be a relevant target for action. Although the strategies mentioned do not show up as short-term changes of state, on the longer term, they help maintain good cell health throughout life.

CHAPTER 8

TARGET 5: AUTOPHAGY

CLEAN YOUR CELLS

What is autophagy and how does it impact health?

You clean your cupboards or desk; you get rid of unuseful or worn out items. And then everything seems less cumbersome and even to work better. For generations, human beings have tried all kinds of approaches to cleanse the body. Even today, companies try to sell you all sorts of supposedly detoxifying or cleansing products. But did you know that the body has a cleaning system of its own and that it kicks in at no cost?

In fact, the body has a number of cleaning systems. One of them we will be examining in greater detail is now being explored by scientists, and its effects on health and longevity seem to be major. It is called autophagy. Autophagy is a "cleaning" system for cells and a "recycling" system for proteins and defective structures that accumulate within cells. This system is generally activated when cells lack energy and raw materials, when they lack "nourishment." During periods of scarcity, this process allows the "waste" that has accumulated inside cells to be destroyed and recovered so that it can be recycled and reused by the body.

As a result, autophagy prevents the accumulation of fats, cleans and protects damaged cells, and activates antioxidizing and anti-inflammatory processes. This process allows the cell to function better, but what is especially interesting is that it also delays cellular senescence and thereby prolongs cell survival. It wasn't without reason that Japanese researcher Yoshinori Ohsumi received the 2016 Nobel Prize in Medicine for his work on autophagy, because, for many specialists, activation of autophagy is an essential ingredient in long healthy life.

What is the impact of inadequate autophagy?

We have seen that some cells renew themselves, while other types of cells remain the same from birth. The latter cell types are particularly sensitive to the accumulation of waste (such as deformed proteins and defective energy systems). As waste accumulates inside the cells, they start to malfunction, and, as discussed below, lay the foundation for certain diseases. The nervous system is made up of cells of this kind. As a result, the brain's functioning and health depend a great deal on effective autophagy. But autophagy has a much greater impact. It is also of capital importance for preserving the capacity of our stem cells, those self-renewing cells, to regenerate healthy tissues and organs.

The activity of the autophagy system tends, however, to diminish with age. For example, the decline in autophagy activity in the dermis as the body ages contributes to making the skin more fragile. Just like skin, the rest of the body is also subject to this age-related slowdown. Over the years, if cellular wastes are not removed, the body is exposed to a variety of diseases, including certain neurodegenerative diseases such as Parkinson's and Alzheimer's. And not only the nervous system can be affected. A less effective cellular cleaning system would favor other conditions and diseases, including:

- lowered resistance to the sun
- atherosclerosis
- cardiovascular diseases
- certain pulmonary diseases
- certain rheumatic diseases

- certain cancers
- muscle loss due to age
- accumulation of fat in the liver

Tools to activate autophagy

The fact that food is so readily available in our industrialized societies allows and even encourages us to respond constantly to the sensation of hunger. A short trip to the fridge or a stop at a drive-in window, and hunger disappears. That is what the ads tell us. Unfortunately, it also prevents the body from activating certain processes that are essential for maintaining long-term health, including autophagy. Moreover, since the autophagy process tends to decline with age, forcing its activation becomes important. Here is how that can be done.

Tool 11. Cut your caloric intake from time to time

How can the cleaning system be activated? According to studies, reducing caloric intake or fasting is THE way to activate the cell cleaning system. As mentioned above, when cells lack energy, they are forced to recycle the waste that they have accumulated. This means that housekeeping is done within the cell, which promotes better cell function. In animal studies, this system is traditionally induced in the liver, brain, and the cells of other tissues by long-term calorie restriction (10% to 30% less) or with 24- to 48-hour fasts. Other studies have shown more concretely that monkeys under calorie restriction developed fewer age-related degenerative diseases and even maintained younger-looking skin. But what is for us the best, simplest, and safest way (i.e. avoiding deficiencies or eating disorders like anorexia) to let the body benefit from a lack of calories? Here are some suggestions:

- Eat less generally, on a daily basis, throughout life. This makes it difficult to avoid nutritional deficiencies, so, in such cases, a recognized nutritional specialist should be consulted.
- Fast for 24 hours once a week or every 2 weeks.
- Reduce your caloric intake by 75% 2 days a week.
- On occasion, (about 5 days per month) choose not to eat lunch and spend at least 16 to 18 consecutive hours without eating.

A number of approaches have been studied and all these strategies, which involve restricting caloric intake, seem to offer some benefit. But because this concept is relatively new to health care, more studies are needed to identify the best strategy. Still, relying on just the studies available now, there can be no doubt that integrating periods of calorie restriction is likely to be a major asset in maintaining long-term health.

If you decide to adopt this approach, however, you should discuss it with your doctor because it could be contraindicated in certain contexts, for example:

- If you are diabetic.
- If you are recovering from an illness or surgery.
- If you have a below-normal body mass index.
- If you are experiencing a growth spurt.
- If you are pregnant, in a preconception period, or breastfeeding.
- If you use medications that have to be taken with food.
- If you want to fast for more than 24 hours.

Although restricting caloric intake is the traditional way of activating autophagy, might there be other ways of achieving the same goal? Others have asked this question; researchers working on it have found some potential solutions.

Giving fasting back a place isn't so hard

For centuries, human beings observed periods of fasting for various reasons, often religious or philosophical. In our industrialized societies, regular (and even constant) intake of food has become the norm. Skipping a meal or two is even considered a cause for concern. "Dr. Minier, you should take the time to eat, it's not good to skip a meal."

Making sure that our friends and family don't go hungry is a form of caring. But, in recent years, more and more studies have shown that fasting has numerous benefits.

The benefits of occasional fasting are first felt in the 5 targets we have established. Besides activating autophagy, calorie restriction activates telomerase and has beneficial antioxidizing, anti-inflammatory, and antiglycating effects. According to animal studies, a reduction in food intake would not only help reach our targets, it would provide an additional benefit in improving stem-cell health. Indeed, it also appears to have a "senolytic" effect, reducing the number of senescent cells in tissues (a mouse study showed that periodically eliminating senescent cells from the body decreased the incidence and slowed the progression of age-related degenerative diseases, which will be revisited below). Certain authors have even suggested that occasional calorie restriction could help destroy cancer cells in tissues in their very early stages. Studies of very large human populations will require many years, but we can already conclude that periods of calorie restriction generate numerous beneficial changes in our bodies. So, there are many arguments for (slowly and harmoniously) adopting this habit.

Fasting must not be considered a penitence or be a hardship. It should be included in daily life with simplicity, as an active health-promoting process. Although the optimum length for gaining the most from calorie restriction has not yet been established, benefits can be felt starting from 18 hours of fasting. While some discomfort may be experienced in the first attempts, the body soon gets used to fasting and such sensations eventually fade away. Starting off with days on which you eat a few foods that are low in calories and have a low glycemic index (e.g., celery, broccoli, cauliflower) can help relief some discomfort and let you gradually get used to fasting. This calorie restriction will probably have little impact on body functions. You will see that, after a few tries, a 24-hour fast is not so hard: you will even feel somewhat lighter!

Tool 12. Resveratrol at the top of the list

Although occasional calorie restriction is an excellent way of taking care of your health and activating the body's cleaning systems, it is not always easy to integrate it into daily life. Some researchers have therefore tried to identify other ways of activating the autophagy system. The result: certain plant extracts have proven to be effective in this regard, and the winner and most thoroughly studied is resveratrol.

In fact, resveratrol is actually the best-known substance for activating the cell cleaning system. Both in vitro and animal studies have shown that consuming resveratrol activates autophagy and extends cell survival. Some authors even suggest that the effect would be felt in dietary doses.

Foods particularly high in resveratrol

- Cranberries
- Lingonberries
- Peanuts
- Pistachios
- Red currants
- Red wine
- Strawberries

Resveratrol is not the only substance that nature offers us to help with cell housekeeping. Another molecule—spermidine—has been clearly identified as triggering this system (see the next page for a list of foods high in spermidine). Spermidine has also been the subject of animal studies, and its consumption has activated cell cleaning systems and enabled animals to live longer. Moreover, resveratrol and spermidine are synergetic when combined (i.e., when they are used together, a smaller quantity of each allows activation of autophagy). Since they have different modes of action, they complement each other in this respect. Another well-known substance—turmeric—acts similarly to spermidine in activating autophagy and, in theory, would work well with resveratrol.

Foods particularly high in spermidine

- Aged cheese
- Corn
- Dried soy beans
- Green peas
- Mushrooms
- Rice bran
- Wheat germ

Because these substances are not easily absorbed by the body and the quantities necessary to activate autophagy have not yet been well established, here is a little tip to maximize resveratrol and turmeric absorption. Piperine, present in pepper, increases the absorption of turmeric by a factor of 20 and that of resveratrol by a factor of 15. It seems that from 10 to 15 mg of piperine (corresponding to about ¼ teaspoon of freshly ground black pepper) per day is enough to benefit from this effect. (*Note: Piperine also increases the absorption of other substances, so it is advisable to discuss this with your doctor or pharmacist, especially if you are taking medications.*)

Tools +. Some other tips

Although these three ingredients (resveratrol, spermidine, and turmeric) are among the most studied activators of autophagy, they are not the only ones. New methods of visualizing autophagy in the body are bringing to light other autophagy activators. First, coffee turns out to be a trigger for the cell cleaning system; four hours after ingesting coffee (regular or decaffeinated), autophagy is activated in the liver, muscles, and heart. Moreover, green tea and physical exertion appear to do the same thing. Finally, consumption of omega-3 fatty acids seems to be a facilitator in activating autophagy.

"Studies have shown that the elimination of senescent cells restores good function to blood vessels and rejuvenates the stem cells in the immune system and muscles."

Tool +. But that's not all...

Research in recent years has revealed a new mechanism that can slow down and even to some extent reverse tissue aging. A mechanism that could be called "senolysis" destroys senescent cells that accumulate in tissues as the individual grows older. As mentioned in Chapter 3, the presence of senescent cells sustains the inflammation that drives accelerated aging. Studies have shown that the elimination of senescent cells restores good function to blood vessels and rejuvenates the stem cells in the immune system and muscles. Another study has shown that, generally, the elimination of these cells postpones the onset of and stabilizes the development of age-related diseases.

With such benefits involved, it's no wonder that pharmaceutical companies are working on this process. Although quercetin (a polyphenol present in cocoa, capers, black elderberries, cloves, red onions, and Mexican oregano) has a senolytic effect, no dosage has been established for this effect. Since this area of study is only in its early stages, the best way to benefit from the senolytic effect is probably to activate autophagy.

So...

Knowledge about autophagy has been growing and suggests that activation of this process has a promising future. The concepts of cell cleaning and senescent-cell disposal are relatively new in the field of health and, in the coming years, they will doubtless assume greater importance. Soon, new laboratory tests will allow real-time visualization of autophagy activation in the human body and we will better understand how to modulate this system. But we already know that this process is very important for preventing age-related diseases, so we don't need to wait to take action.

CHAPTER 9

STRATEGY REVIEW: PUTTING THE JIGSAW PUZZLE BACK TOGETHER

Before going further, let's take a moment to consolidate what has been discussed up to this point. Everything we do is designed to obtain a benefit, and reading this book is no exception. We have noted a major problem in our industrialized societies: health deteriorates with age, but it is quite clear that this problem can be avoided. Research was performed and scientific articles selected in writing this book with the goal of obtaining 3 specific benefits for avoiding this problem and keeping future generations from being exposed to needless aging. The benefits sought are:

1. **Maintaining function as long as possible:** muscle strength, an immune system in good working order, visual acuity, a keen mind, memory, sexual function, etc.
2. **Postponing the appearance of age-related diseases:** Alzheimer's disease, stroke, osteoporosis, etc.
3. **Reduce overall cancer risks.**

As we have seen, the body's health requires that cells be maintained in good condition. The targets and tools described herein have been the subject of scientific studies and each has an essential place in this general strategy, like pieces in a jigsaw puzzle. Achieving the targets described and using the tools presented in this book will enable the body to fully apply the important steps that contribute to preventing cells and tissues from aging. These steps are:

Step 1: Prevent genotoxic and cytotoxic stress.

As in many cases, prevention is the keystone to long-term health. Preventing damage to the genetic code (genotoxic stress) and cell components (cytotoxic stress) is therefore the foundation. Most of the targets described in this book are intended to have a preventive effect: containing excess oxidation (Chapter 4), overcoming chronic inflammation (Chapter 5), avoiding glycation (Chapter 6), and preserving telomeres (Chapter 7) are our main targets; prevention tools are described in each of these chapters.

Step 2: Repair and clean cell structures.

Although we are improving the odds for protecting our cells, the environment ultimately causes damage either to cell components or the genetic code. Repairing this damage and cleaning the structures that cannot be repaired are also vital for maintaining healthy and well-functioning cells.

First, in case of *damage to cellular structures,* the repair systems activate themselves, but we don't know much about how to stimulate this mechanism. Damaged structures can also be destroyed and recycled. The preferred method for doing this, as described in Chapter 8, is activating autophagy, which is essential for maintaining long-term health.

Then, if the cell's *genetic code is damaged*, the DNA repair systems must go into action. This process is important at all times for all the cells in the body. We have not discussed DNA repair very much but some substances found in food have shown a potential for activating the genetic-code repair system. Some foods that have demonstrated a capacity to stimulate repairs to the genetic code of cells are grape-seed oil; green-tea polyphenols; honey; and rosmarinic acid, which occurs in rosemary but also in basil, lemon balm, sage, thyme, and marjoram, among other herbs.

Step 3: Eliminate senescent cells.

Lastly, despite the optimization of the prevention and repair processes, certain cells will have been altered too much and become senescent. As seen above, the accumulation of senescent cells promotes inflammation in tissues. Their periodic elimination has demonstrated benefits in delaying the appearance and stabilizing the development of age-related diseases, and even reversing damage to certain tissues. Activation of the senolytic process is therefore a good idea, at least occasionally, to keep the body young and healthy (Chapter 8).

So, the simple tools I have described are to be used throughout life, starting in youth. They will enable us to directly affect our cells and help them continue to work properly, which will promote maintaining our own quality of life and that of our children on the long term.

CHAPTER 10

DERMATOLOGIST SPECIAL: CARING FOR YOUR SKIN FROM THE INSIDE OUT

———

Why not spend a little time on your skin? After all, our starting point was the fact that areas of skin may age faster and others slower. Because skin cells behave the same way as other body cells, skin health is not unrelated to an individual's general state of health. In one study, researchers evaluated the condition of the skin in an area unexposed to the sun, like the inner thigh. They were able to show that, at comparable ages, less wrinkled skin was associated with better health and, conversely, people with more wrinkles had poorer health. So, taking care of health holistically can only benefit the skin. Generally speaking, trying to reach our five targets will have benefits for skin health. But why shouldn't I, as a dermatologist, before concluding, share a few tips discovered in the medical literature that could more specifically contribute to improving the appearance and health of skin.

First, and this has been clearly demonstrated, there is a link between wrinkles, skin cancers, and ultraviolet exposure. These rays are the primary cause of accelerated skin aging. This is well known because these rays are major generators of oxidative stress and inflammation, our first two targets. As mentioned at the beginning of this book, these processes damage DNA (the genetic code), shorten telomeres, and push cells toward senescence. The skin then begins to work less effectively: collagen diminishes, the skin dries out more easily and its color becomes irregular, blood vessels become more fragile, and cells are at greater risk of transforming into cancer cells.

Certain well-known basic rules can help prevent the skin from aging. First, exposure to the sun's ultraviolet rays should be limited by avoiding peak hours, wearing protective clothing (and protective eyewear), and, as a last resort, using sunscreen. As mentioned in previous chapters, it is also important for skin health to avoid other factors that damage cells (smoking, atmospheric pollution, etc.).

Lastly, getting adequate sleep and taking adequate hormone supplements (when indicated) will also contribute to keeping skin in better health.

But can we expect our dietary choices to affect skin health? The answer is unhesitatingly yes! Our dietary choices influence the skin both generally and specifically, acting as "protective tools" for skin health. Here are a few tips.

Arm your body against the sun

As a dermatologist, I find myself saying this every day: skin must be protected in order to reduce needless aging caused by the sun. According to some studies, however, certain foods may reduce the risk of sunburn. Here are some of them. First, generally speaking, a diet high in omega-3 fatty acids would appear to be beneficial in improving sun tolerance. More specifically, other foods have demonstrated benefits, including dark chocolate and tea (high in polyphenols). Foods cooked with tomato paste also deserve mention, since regular consumption of tomato paste appears to reduce sunburn sensitivity and may also protect DNA against damage caused by ultraviolet rays. In fact, an extract of a type of fern called *polypodium leucotomos* (240 mg twice a day) can also reduce sun sensitivity, the risk of sunburn, and skin damage caused by sun exposure. Lastly, drinking a glass of red wine (high in polyphenols) prior to ultraviolet exposure can also reduce the risk of sunburn!

"But can we expect our dietary choices to affect skin health? The answer is unhesitatingly yes!'

Reducing the risks of skin cancer

Since the incidence of skin cancer has been constantly rising and the disease affects people at ever younger ages, we need to do everything possible to reduce its risks and consequences. Of course, adopting good sun habits is important. But, like with sun tolerance, certain foods can reduce the risk of developing skin cancer. First, a diet high in fruits and vegetables has been associated with a lower risk of developing skin cancer. As for specific foods, coffee (not the decaffeinated kind), wine, and tea appear to offer some protection. Lastly, taking fish-oil or grape-seed-oil supplements may also be helpful in reducing the risks of developing a skin cancer.

Maintaining beautiful skin

Cosmetic ads promising softer skin with more homogeneous color and texture abound. While anti-aging creams often improve the skin's appearance, good lifestyle habits have a more profound effect on skin function and cell aging. A healthy body generates skin that is healthy and more homogeneous overall and that tends to wrinkle less quickly. Here again, certain specific foods have shown benefits in preserving beautiful skin, and some tips really should be emphasized. First, a study showed that participants taking *Lactobacillus plantarum* supplements for 3 months had improved hydration and their skin was more glowing and less wrinkled than that of their counterparts receiving a placebo. Twelve-week studies in which participants consumed chocolate high in polyphenols, green tea, or Asian ginseng extracts demonstrated a benefit in improving skin texture and hydration. Consumption of olive oil (monosaturated fat), omega-3 fatty acids, and *moderate* amounts of alcohol was associated with a reduction in signs of sun aging. In another study, menopausal women taking a soy extract showed improvements in the appearance of wrinkles and an increase in collagen after 3 to 6 months. Red-clover isoflavones also seemed to have a beneficial effect. Lastly, the lycopene (found in tomatoes, watermelon, papaya, guava, and pink grapefruit) in the skin seems to produce softer skin.

And what about those anti-wrinkle creams?

On store shelves, touted in ads, and featured in magazine articles: anti-wrinkle creams are everywhere. Their virtues are equaled only by the imagination used by advertising agencies in vaunting their merits. Even though they are everywhere, we would do well to take a moment to examine this phenomenon and their anti-aging potential.

First, remember that the processes that accelerate skin aging are the same as those involved in the body's aging: our 5 targets! More specifically, from the dermatology point of view, exposure to the sun and ultraviolet rays plays a major role in skin aging. Moreover, smoking clearly contributes to the aging of dermis and epidermis cells. Furthermore, hormonal changes also play a role, given the decline in skin's water-retention capacity and a loss of 30% of collagen in the 5 years after menopause. The basic approach is to maintain good sun habits, good lifestyle habits in reaching our 5 goals, and perhaps a hormone supplement. There is no consensus in the literature about the benefits for the skin of taking hormone supplements; you should discuss this with your doctor.

As for hydrating creams, dry skin becomes inflamed more easily, so applying a hydrating agent can be beneficial. Generally, a hydrating cream containing a few basic ingredients will do the job. In addition, the hydration provided by a cream is enough to make the skin appear less wrinkled and less dull. So, there is no need spend a lot of money to achieve good hydration and restore a bit of tone to dried-out skin.

Of course, some companies claim that their products deliver special advantages. True, some creams can exfoliate, reduce brown spots, or even slightly boost collagen production. Yet if you really want to be reassured of a product's benefits—regardless of the active ingredients it contains (antioxidant, vitamin, stem cells, etc.)—look for evidence that the benefit has been demonstrated in a study that compares the active cream to a placebo cream. Studies that show results before and after the cream has been applied are generally not enough to warrant the product's higher cost. As for slowing aging, although some creams may offer a slight benefit, the strategies mentioned above remain the best investment.

So, that's the story!

Achieving our 5 targets keeps our cells healthy and allows the body to function better for years. But these strategies also help the skin by improving its resistance to all attackers, even those we have very little control over, such as atmospheric pollution. These strategies therefore reduce the risks of developing cancer and keep skin looking younger for longer. There you have it: another good reason for adopting healthy habits!

CHAPTER 11

IN CLOSING: MARKETING THE FOUNTAIN OF YOUTH

—

Illness is costly: doctor's visits, surgical procedures, medications, downtime. Modern medicine has developed increasingly effective ways of dealing with health problems. Long-term studies have established the efficacy and safety of these tools, which contribute to increasing the cost of treatments. But what about the costs for preventing aging? What should we choose among the many offerings that are intended to prolong youth?

"As seen above, high doses of antioxidants can be harmful by preventing certain of the body's processes from working properly."

A scientist who graduated from X University has just developed a test to identify what you should avoid eating to get back your energy. An Internet "doctor" offers a fantastic product made from stem cells that, because of its epigenetic action, will allow your cells to be reprogrammed as if you were 25 years old. The Fountain of Youth market is enormous. Many companies try to take advantage of our fear of aging by touting the magical results of a product or approach that relieves us of being responsible for our own health. The aging process is complex. No supplement, no matter how revolutionary, can restore the body to a state of optimal balance to prolong health. Moreover, supplements may present risks. As seen above, high doses of antioxidants can be harmful by preventing certain of the body's processes from working properly. As things stand, we clearly know which supplements are needed such as iodine in table salt, and calcium and vitamin D in official recommendations. But there is no miracle supplement looming on the horizon!

In the future, we may be able to reprogram cells and maintain them as they were when we were 20 years old. But that's not today's reality and, of course, if it happens, it will come with a price tag. For the time being, good habits are our best allies, and the strategies for reaching our 5 targets don't cost anything. Don't get misled by people peddling the Fountain of Youth. If you want to invest money in maintaining your health, invest it in what gives pleasure to you and your loved ones. That is an excellent investment in your health.

CONCLUSION

———

In this book, I have pointed out a number of effective (and free) strategies for activating the right processes that help prevent aging, degenerative diseases, and certain cancers. This involves 5 targets: preventing oxidation, preventing inflammation, preventing glycation, activating autophagy, and activating telomerase. These are probably the most relevant targets for maintaining long-term health, that is, the health of our youth. Some strategies hit 1 or 2 targets; others strike all 5 at once. For example, including the habit of physical exercise is another strategy that reaches all 5 targets. Likewise, adding herbs and spices to food before cooking and even on the plate is another way of hitting several targets, and it is a very easy strategy to implement, at that. Herbs and spices are concentrates of anti-aging process activators. Of course, the body needs quality food in sufficient quantities to rebuild and *regenerate* itself, but periods for cleaning are also essential. As mentioned, restricting caloric intake on an occasional basis activates these cleaning processes and provides numerous other benefits for the whole body. And these are only some of the tools that are easy to begin including in your life.

"But, as doctors, we are only starting to recognize the importance of activating the processes that protect the body against aging.

As doctors, my colleagues and I encounter patients every day: we know only too well that despite adopting good habits, a person's health sometimes doesn't cooperate. Treating diseases remains an important way of enabling people to maintain a better quality of life and live longer. By doing so, we still help extend life expectancy. But when it comes to extending health expectancy, medical treatment won't do the trick. It is the labor of a lifetime.

As doctors, we encourage our patients to adopt good habits: avoid smoking, limit sun exposure, cut down on salt, avoid refined sugars, follow the recommendations of the food guides, and more. But, as doctors, we are only starting to recognize the importance of activating the processes that protect the body against aging. These protective tools help us defend ourselves against the harmful aggressors we know and maybe against those we don't yet know in maintaining the health of all of our organs. As noted earlier, aging doesn't cause any symptoms. No alarm goes off for either the patient or the doctor, motivating them to take action. Taking action, however, is essential before arriving at a fait accompli and having to admit: "I've gotten old."

We therefore have to move contrary to certain elements that our industrialized society fosters: the various electronic displays leading us to increasingly sedentary lives, the refined diet that deprives our intestinal flora of essential nutrients, the abundance of foods that satisfy hunger as soon as it is felt... These solutions that make daily life easier are presented as a kind of societal evolution. In fact, however, they are the opposite of what the body needs to live long and healthy. As seen above, they generate an imbalance through excess oxidation, excess inflammation, and accumulated waste in body cells. The strategies described herein help fight these phenomena and contribute to maintaining better health for many years.

One day, a 99-year-old patient told me: "Daniel, I'm getting older, but I'm not aging." He was unhappy because his 80-year-old friends were too old for him! And I realized he was right: getting older without aging is possible. It starts young, during intrauterine life, and it continues day by day. Yet it's never too late to start, because reaching certain targets lets the body function the way it did when it was (a little) younger. Taking charge of your life, as an individual and family, and incorporating anti-aging habits can be done step-by-step; the tools are there and they work.

Don't run the risk of aging: pick your tools and get started.

DR. DANIEL MINIER

Q AND A

———

I find intermittent fasting very hard. What is the simplest way of obtaining the benefits of calorie restriction?

The most honest answer is: we don't yet know. In the future, new laboratory tests will teach us more about the simplest ways of activating autophagy, one of the systems essential for maintaining long-term health. While seeking the minimum effort for reaching this objective, we can already suggest some answers, based on a few studies, as follows.

First, researchers asked a group of people to allocate their caloric intake differently. For 2 weeks, the intake was divided up differently on alternate days: one day, 25% of their normal daily caloric intake; the next, 175% of their daily caloric intake. After 3 weeks, the same number of calories had been ingested, but it was possible to detect an onset of activation of the genes associated with autophagy.

Second, a nightly fast of more than 13 hours might play a role in reducing the risk of relapse in women survivors of breast cancer. Moreover, if this type of fasting was extended to about 16 hours, additional benefits could be observed regarding insulin resistance and inflammation.

So, even rather short fasts reap certain benefits. But remember that a good meal always has its place in maintaining good health. The benefits of this type of fasting tend to be observed mainly in people who stop their caloric intake in the evening, after 5 p.m.

Wegman MP, Guo MH, Bennion DM, Shankar MN, Chrzanowski SM, Goldberg LA, Xu J, Williams TA, Lu X, Hsu SI, Anton SD, Leeuwenburgh C, Brantly ML. Practicality of intermittent fasting in humans and its effect on oxidative stress and genes related to aging and metabolism. Rejuvenation Res. 2015 Apr;18(2):162-72.

Brad Kincaid, Ella Bossy-Wetzel. Forever young: SIRT3 a shield against mitochondrial meltdown, aging, and neurodegeneration. Front Aging Neurosci. 2013; 5: 48.

Marinac CR, Nelson SH, Breen CI, Hartman SJ, Natarajan L, Pierce JP, Flatt SW, Sears DD, Patterson RE. Prolonged Nightly Fasting and Breast Cancer Prognosis. JAMA Oncol. 2016 Aug 1;2(8):1049-55.

Bi H, Gan Y, Yang C, Chen Y, Tong X, Lu Z. Breakfast skipping and the risk of type 2 diabetes: a meta-analysis of observational studies. Public Health Nutr. 2015 Nov;18(16):3013-9.

Catherine R. Marinac, Dorothy D. Sears, Loki Natarajan, Linda C. Gallo, Caitlin I. Breen, Ruth E. Patterson. Frequency and Circadian Timing of Eating May Influence Biomarkers of Inflammation and Insulin Resistance Associated with Breast Cancer Risk. PLoS One. 2015; 10(8): e0136240.

Are there tips for not feeling too hungry when fasting?

First of all, practice; it seems that people who fast occasionally eventually get used to it, and their system learns to manage the lack of calories.

According to a study, L-carnitine supplements might reduce the feeling of hunger and fatigue associated with fasting. This study, however, used intravenous infusion of L-carnitine.

Finally, as mentioned earlier, a fast must not be considered a punishment. It is probable, in my opinion, that having a cup of coffee or herbal tea, or a few low-calorie vegetables (celery, cauliflower, etc.) would not interfere with the benefits of calorie restriction.

Zhang JJ, Wu ZB, Cai YJ, Ke B, Huang YJ, Qiu CP, Yang YB, Shi LY, Qin J.L-carnitine ameliorated fasting-induced fatigue, hunger, and metabolic abnormalities in patients with metabolic syndrome: a randomized controlled study. Nutr J. 2014 Nov 26;13:110.

If I have understood you correctly, grilled meat is not very good for your health, but I enjoy the meals my husband prepares on the BBQ. Do you have a solution for him?

You have correctly understood that cooking on the grill generates the formation of advanced glycation end products (which cause inflammation throughout the body) as well as the formation of heterocyclic amines (toxic for the genetic code).

The consequences of advanced glycation end products (AGEs) were laid out in Chapter 6, but let's look at the effects of ingesting heterocyclic amines (HCAs). First of all, heterocyclic amines in the digestive system could contribute to developing colon cancer. In addition, the toxic products of grilled meat could contribute to developing bladder cancer. Lastly, for men, the more grilled or well-done red meat they eat, the more of these toxic products that accumulate in the prostate and the higher the risk of having an aggressive prostate cancer. How to avoid these effects?

The first option is not to grill or roast meat. But if you really love your barbecue, there are three ways of reducing the formation and mitigating the harmful effects of these toxic products.

Tip No. 1: ADD SPICES. A study compared two meatballs: one with and one without a mixture of herbs and spices. Once cooked, the seasoned meatball had less of the toxic products. Moreover, the urine of people who had eaten the seasoned meatball contained half as many of these toxic products.

Tip No. 2: USE MARINADES. As described in Chapter 6, marinating meat in vinegar reduces the formation of AGEs while providing a supplementary benefit. One study has shown that using a marinade (for several hours) made of beer or vinegar as well as herbs and spices reduces the formation of HCAs by more than 90%. This protection seems effective for up to 30 minutes of cooking. After 40 or more minutes on the grill, no benefit was obtained.

Tip No. 3: SOCIALIZE. Researchers measured the quantity of HCAs in human prostates. They asked these men about what they drank, and, of 15 beverages evaluated, only red wine (probably because of its resveratrol content; see Chapter 7) was associated with a low rate of HCAs in the prostate.

Note: If you are the parent of teenagers, you should know that eating red meat during adolescence increases the risk of breast cancer as an adult.

Bouvard, Véronique et al. Carcinogenicity of consumption of red and processed meat The Lancet Oncology , Volume 16 , Issue 16 , 1599 - 1600

Lee DH, Keum N, Giovannucci EL. Colorectal Cancer Epidemiology in the Nurses' Health Study. Am J Public Health. 2016 Sep;106(9):1599-607.

Lin J, Forman MR, Wang J, Grossman HB, Chen M, Dinney CP, Hawk ET, Wu X.Intake of red meat and heterocyclic amines, metabolic pathway genes and bladder cancer risk. Int J Cancer. 2012 Oct 15;131(8):1892-903

Li F, An S, Hou L, Chen P, Lei C, Tan W. Red and processed meat intake and risk of bladder cancer: a meta-analysis. Int J Clin Exp Med. 2014 Aug 15;7(8):2100-10. eCollection 2014.

Tang D, Liu JJ, Rundle A, Neslund-Dudas C, Savera AT, Bock CH, Nock NL, Yang JJ, Rybicki BA. Grilled meat consumption and PhIP-DNA adducts in prostate carcinogenesis. Cancer Epidemiol Biomarkers Prev. 2007 Apr;16(4):803-8.

John EM, Stern MC, Sinha R, Koo J. Meat consumption, cooking practices, meat mutagens, and risk of prostate cancer. Nutr Cancer. 2011;63(4):525-37.

Li Z, Henning SM, Zhang Y, Zerlin A, Li L, Gao K, Lee RP, Karp H, Thames G, Antioxidant-rich spice added to hamburger meat during cooking results in reduced meat, plasma, and urine malondialdehyde concentrations. Am J Clin Nutr. 2010 May;91(5):1180-4.

Melo A, Viegas O, Petisca C, Pinho O, Ferreira IM. Effect of beer/red wine marinades on the formation of heterocyclic aromatic amines in pan-fried beef. J Agric Food Chem. 2008 Nov 26;56(22):10625-32.

Salmon CP, Knize MG, Felton JS. Effects of marinating on heterocyclic amine carcinogen formation in grilled chicken. Food Chem Toxicol. 1997 May;35(5):433-41.

Rybicki BA, Neslund-Dudas C, Bock CH, Nock NL, Rundle A, Jankowski M, Levin AM, Beebe-Dimmer J, Savera AT, Takahashi S, Shirai T, Tang D. Red wine consumption is inversely associated with 2-amino-1-methyl-6-phenylimidazo[4,5-b]pyridine-DNA adduct levels in prostate. Cancer Prev Res (Phila). 2011 Oct;4(10):1636-44.

Farvid MS, Cho E, Chen WY, Eliassen AH, Willett WC. Adolescent meat intake and breast cancer risk. Int J Cancer. 2015 Apr 15;136(8):1909-20.

I have read elsewhere that alcohol can increase your life expectancy, but you didn't mention that in this book.

The impact of alcohol is rather complex and cannot be included in an overall aging-prevention strategy. Generally speaking, although drinking red wine in light to moderate quantities (about 1 glass a day for women and 2 for men) seems to improve life expectancy by about 5 years, it generates an "exchange" of cause of mortality. The cardiovascular benefits are obtained at the cost of an increase in certain types of cancers. There is no safe level of drinking for certain cancers, that is, from the first glass, the risk of developing certain cancers (e.g. liver, mouth, throat, esophagus, breast) begins to rise. Alcohol therefore does not replace an anti-aging strategy. At best, it can be added, prudently and avoiding certain harmful behaviors.

If you don't drink alcohol, don't start now: there are other, safer strategies.

Don't exceed the quantities mentioned, because the benefits are quickly exceeded by the risks (cancers, stroke, ischemic heart disease, diabetes, obesity).

Binge drinking should be avoided at all costs. Such episodes, even if infrequent, can have harmful effects on your health.

If you tend to be alcohol dependent, if you find it hard to limit your consumption, or if alcohol modifies your behavior in a way that is harmful to you or those around you, the best strategy is to avoid drinking alcohol and opt for nonalcoholic beverages instead.

Yue Zhou, Jie Zheng, Sha Li, Tong Zhou, Pei Zhang, Hua-Bin Li. Alcoholic Beverage Consumption and Chronic Diseases. Int J Environ Res Public Health. 2016 Jun; 13(6): 522.

Yin Cao, Walter C Willett, Eric B Rimm, Meir J Stampfer, Edward L Giovannucci, Light to moderate intake of alcohol, drinking patterns, and risk of cancer: results from two prospective US cohort studies. BMJ. 2015; 351: h4238.

Roerecke M1, Rehm J. Alcohol consumption, drinking patterns, and ischemic heart disease: a narrative review of meta-analyses and a systematic review and meta-analysis of the impact of heavy drinking occasions on risk for moderate drinkers. BMC Med. 2014 Oct 21;12:182.

Streppel MT, Ocké MC, Boshuizen HC, Kok FJ, Kromhout D. Long-term wine consumption is related to cardiovascular mortality and life expectancy independently of moderate alcohol intake: the Zutphen Study. J Epidemiol Community Health. 2009 Jul;63(7):534-40.

What is the role of hormone supplements in staying healthy at an advanced age?

The decline in hormone levels observed with age seems to be associated with the appearance of certain age-related problems (frail skin, osteoporosis, alteration of sexual function, etc.). Some studies show real benefits for quality of life, but others warn against potential risks. Given these studies, some doctors reject hormone supplements out of hand as a way of maintaining quality of life on the long term, while others see them as nearly a fountain of youth. In my opinion, the truth lies somewhere between the two, with a benefit in favor of hormone supplementation started as soon as symptoms of deficiency begin.

With an aging population, new studies will make it possible to clarify what the realistic expectations should be and what types of hormones are most beneficial and safe. Since there are certain contraindications to taking hormone supplements, this decision must be considered after an evaluation and discussion with a health-care professional. Hormone supplementation, however, will not replace lifestyle habits and must be part of an overall strategy for maintaining long-term health.

NICE Guideline, No. 23. Long-term benefits and risks of hormone replacement therapy (HRT) National Collaborating Centre for Women's and Children's Health (UK). London: National Institute for Health and Care Excellence (UK); 2015 Nov 12.

Hackett GI. Testosterone Replacement Therapy and Mortality in Older Men. Drug Saf. 2016 Feb;39(2):117-30.

Why should I worry about my habits now if, in the future, we will be able to regenerate my organs from stem cells?

Regenerative medicine will represent a major step in the treatment of many health problems, including those related to age. These strategies, however, are still beyond our reach and many challenges remain to be met.

But there is one even more important element to consider: the brain! Memory, memories, and personality—the elements that contribute to defining a person as an individual—are forged by the connection of billions of neurons. Each and every one of us has a different neural network.

Although new stem cells are formed in the brain, it is unlikely that one stem cell will be able to replace, with all the same connections, the neurons that already exist in the brain.

So, again, the most reliable approach for now is to prevent the needless aging of tissues. This will simultaneously maintain neurons, stem cells, and their niche or environment in good condition. And, if we live long enough to witness the advent of regenerative medicine, we and our children will have done everything we can to optimize the success rates of this approach.

Kusumbe AP, Ramasamy SK, Itkin T, Mäe MA, Langen UH, Betsholtz C, Lapidot T, Adams RH. Age-dependent modulation of vascular niches for haematopoietic stem cells. Nature. 2016 Apr 21;532(7599):380-4.

Singh L, Brennan TA, Russell E, Kim JH, Chen Q, Brad Johnson F, Pignolo RJ. Aging alters bone-fat reciprocity by shifting in vivo mesenchymal precursor cell fate towards an adipogenic lineage. Bone. 2016 Apr;85:29-36.

Mendelson A, Frenette PS. Hematopoietic stem cell niche maintenance during homeostasis and regeneration. Nat Med. 2014 Aug;20(8):833-46. doi: 10.1038/nm.3647.

Maximina H. Yun. Changes in Regenerative Capacity through Lifespan. Int J Mol Sci. 2015 Oct; 16(10): 25392-25432.

Wrinkles, skin cancer, vitamin D...Is there any way to have safe sun?

There is no doubt that exposure to ultraviolet rays, whether from the sun or tanning beds, causes cancer and premature aging of the skin. My patients who have spent long hours outdoors during their lives present with numerous precancerous and cancerous lesions, mainly on the face, in addition to wrinkles and brown spots. Others, who work mainly indoors, are at greater risk of developing melanomas, a form of cancer principally associated with sunburn.

So, sun protection is without question appropriate. First, exposure should be limited during peak hours of sunlight (between 10 a.m. and 2 p.m.). Then, protective clothing should be worn, ideally even while swimming (there are very nice rash guards as well as sunglasses). And lastly, apply sunscreens to the areas exposed to the sun. Sunscreens are used as a last resort because their absorption by the body presents a not-yet-much-studied potential to disrupt the function of certain cells and genetic material. Moreover, these products wind up in the environment and may pollute watercourses.

There are also benefits of exposing the skin to sunlight. The best-known benefit is, of course, vitamin D, which is produced by the skin exposed to UVB rays. Supplements can be used to compensate, but the skin can produce other useful molecules under the effect of sunlight. Vitamin D, however, is not the sun's only benefit for skin. Studies have shown that sunlight also has a beneficial effect on blood pressure, multiple sclerosis, and rheumatoid arthritis.

And lastly, although sunburns promote the development of melanoma, a **little** exposure to sunlight without sunburn at any age appears to have a protective effect on the incidence and severity of melanomas.

So, wise use of the sun appears to be finding a balance between good protection and some exposure. In any case, activating natural protective mechanisms (see Chapters 9 and 11) appears to be additional protection against cancer as much as against accelerated aging.

Ramos S. et coll. A review of organic UV-filters in wastewater treatment plants. Environ Int. 2016 Jan;86:24-44. doi: 10.1016/j.envint.2015.10.004

Louis GM. Et coll. Urinary concentrations of benzophenone-type ultraviolet light filters and semen quality. Fertil Steril. 2015 Oct;104(4):989-96. doi: 10.1016/j.fertnstert.2015.07.1129.

Nicole Bijlsma, Marc M. Cohen. Environmental Chemical Assessment in Clinical Practice: Unveiling the Elephant in the Room Int J Environ Res Public Health. 2016 Feb; 13(2): 181.

Narayanan KB et al. Disruptive environmental chemicals and cellular mechanisms that confer resistance to cell death. Carcinogenesis. 2015 Jun;36 Suppl 1:S89-110.

Slominski A et al. Novel vitamin D photoproducts and their precursors in the skin. Dermatoendocrinol. 2013 Jan 1;5(1):7-19.

Liu D et al. UVA Irradiation of Human Skin Vasodilates Arterial Vasculature and Lowers Blood Pressure Independently of Nitric Oxide Synthase. J Invest Dermatol. 2014 Jan 20. doi: 10.1038/jid.2014.27.

Arkema EV et al. Exposure to ultraviolet-B and risk of developing rheumatoid arthritis among women in the Nurses' Health Study. Ann Rheum Dis. 2013 Apr;72(4):506-11. doi: 10.1136/annrheumdis-2012-202302. Epub 2013 Feb 4.

William B. Grant. The role of geographical ecological studies in identifying diseases linked to UVB exposure and/or vitamin D. Dermatoendocrinol. 2016 Jan-Dec; 8(1): e1137400.

Asta Juzeniene , Johan Moan. Beneficial effects of UV radiation other than via vitamin D production. Dermatoendocrinol. 2012 April 1; 4(2): 109–117.

Kaskel P et al. Outdoor activities in childhood: a protective factor for cutaneous melanoma? Results of a case-control study in 271 matched pairs. Br J Dermatol. 2001 Oct;145(4):602-9.

Gandini S. et cal. Sun exposure and melanoma prognostic factors. Oncol Lett. 2016 Apr;11(4):2706-2714.

Newton-Bishop JA. et al. Relationship between sun exposure and melanoma risk for tumours in different body sites in a large case-control study in a temperate climate. Eur J Cancer. 2011 Mar;47(5):732-41. doi: 10.1016/j.ejca.2010.10.008.

SOME OF THE REFERENCES

GENERAL

Website of Institut national de la statistique et des études économiques : http://www.insee.fr/fr/themes/tableau.asp?ref_id=CMPECF02228

Dong X, Milholland B, Vijg J.Evidence for a limit to human lifespan. Nature. 2016 Oct 5;538(7624):257-259.

SENESCENCE

Race DiLoreto, Coleen T. Murphy. The cell biology of aging. Mol Biol Cell. 2015 Dec 15; 26(25): 4524–4531.

Naina Bhatia-Dey, Riya R. Kanherkar, Susan E. Stair,Evgeny O. Makarev, Antonei B. Csoka.Cellular Senescence as the Causal Nexus of Aging. Front Genet. 2016; 7: 13.

Adams PD, Jasper H, Rudolph KL. Aging-Induced Stem Cell Mutations as Drivers for Disease and Cancer. Cell Stem Cell. 2015 Jun 4;16(6):601-12.

Ruhland MK, Loza AJ, Capietto AH, Luo X, Knolhoff BL, Flanagan KC, Belt BA, Alspach E, Leahy K, Luo J, Schaffer A, Edwards JR,Longmore G, Faccio R3, DeNardo DG, Stewart SA. Stromal senescence establishes an immunosuppressive microenvironment that drives tumorigenesis. Nat Commun. 2016 Jun 8;7:11762.

Finkel, Toren, Serrano, Manuel, Blasco, Maria A. The common biology of cancer and ageing. Nature. Volume 448(7155), 16 August 2007, pp 767-774

Tchkonia T, Morbeck DE, Von Zglinicki T, Van Deursen J, Lustgarten J, Scrable H, Khosla S, Jensen MD, Kirkland JL. Fat tissue, aging, and cellular senescence. Aging Cell. 2010 Oct;9(5):667-84.

Feng C, Liu H, Yang M, Zhang Y, Huang B, Zhou Y. Disc cell senescence in intervertebral disc degeneration: Causes and molecular pathways. Cell Cycle. 2016 Jul 2;15(13):1674-84.

Davalos AR, Coppe JP, Campisi J, Desprez PY. Senescent cells as a source of inflammatory factors for tumor progression. Cancer Metastasis Rev. 2010 Jun;29(2):273-83.

Tzyy Yue Wong, Mairim Alexandra Solis, Ying-Hui Chen, Lynn Ling-Huei Huang Molecular mechanism of extrinsic factors affecting anti-aging of stem cells. World J Stem Cells. 2015 Mar 26; 7(2): 512-520.

López-Otín C, Blasco MA, Partridge L, Serrano M, Kroemer G. The hallmarks of aging. Cell. 2013 Jun 6;153(6):1194-217.

OXYDATIVE STRESS

Jimenez-Del-Rio M, Velez-Pardo C. The bad, the good, and the ugly about oxidative stress. 2012;2012:163913.

Araujo JA. Particulate air pollution, systemic oxidative stress, inflammation, and atherosclerosis. Air Qual Atmos Health. 2010 Nov 10;4(1):79-93.

Piskounova E, Agathocleous M, Murphy MM, Hu Z, Huddlestun SE, Zhao Z, Leitch AM, Johnson TM, DeBerardinis RJ, Morrison SJ. Oxidative stress inhibits distant metastasis by human melanoma cells. Nature. 2015 Nov 12;527(7577):186-91.

Bjelakovic G, Nikolova D, Gluud LL, Simonetti RG, Gluud C. Antioxidant supplements for prevention of mortality in healthy participants and patients with various diseases. Cochrane Database Syst Rev. 2012 Mar 14;(3):CD007176. doi: 10.1002/14651858.CD007176.pub2.

INFLAMMATION

Puzianowska-Kuźnicka M, Owczarz M, Wieczorowska-Tobis K, Nadrowski P, Chudek J, Slusarczyk P, Skalska A, Jonas M, Franek E,Mossakowska M. Interleukin-6 and C-reactive protein, successful aging, and mortality: the PolSenior study. Immun Ageing. 2016 Jun 3;13:21.

Minciullo PL, Catalano A, Mandraffino G, Casciaro M, Crucitti A, Maltese G, Morabito N, Lasco A, Gangemi S, Basile G. Inflammaging and Anti-Inflammaging: The Role of Cytokines in Extreme Longevity. Arch Immunol Ther Exp (Warsz). 2016 Apr;64(2):111-26.

O'Donovan A, Neylan TC, Metzle T, Cohen BE. Lifetime exposure to traumatic psychological stress is associated with elevated inflammation in the Heart and Soul Study. Brain Behav Immun. 2012 May;26(4):642-9.

Bruno Deltreggia Benites, Simone Cristina Olenscki Gilli, Sara Teresinha Olalla Saad Obesity and inflammation and the effect on the hematopoietic system. Rev Bras Hematol Hemoter. 2014 Mar-Apr; 36(2): 147-151.

André C, Dinel AL, Ferreira G, Layé S, Castanon N. Diet-induced obesity progressively alters cognition, anxiety-like behavior and lipopolysaccharide-induced depressive-like behavior: focus on brain indoleamine 2,3-dioxygenase activation.brain Behav Immun. 2014 Oct;41:10-21.

Castanon N, Lasselin J, Capuron L. Neuropsychiatric comorbidity in obesity: role of inflammatory processes. Front Endocrinol (Lausanne). 2014 May 15;5:74.

George M. Slavich, Michael R. Irwin. From Stress to Inflammation and Major Depressive Disorder: A Social Signal Transduction Theory of Depression. Psychol Bull. May 2014; 140(3): 774-815.

Anders S, Tanaka M, Kinney DK. Depression as an evolutionary strategy for defense against infection. Brain Behav Immun. 2013 Jul;31:9-22.

Raison CL, Miller AH. Malaise, melancholia and madness: the evolutionary legacy of an inflammatory bias. Brain Behav Immun. 2013 Jul;31:1-8.

Miquel-Kergoat S, Azais-Braesco V, Burton-Freeman B, Hetherington MM. Effects of chewing on appetite, food intake and gut hormones: A systematic review and meta-analysis. Physiol Behav. 2015 Nov 1;151:88-96.

Cho HJ, Kivimäki M, Bower JE, Irwin MR. Association of C-reactive protein and interleukin-6 with new-onset fatigue in the Whitehall II prospective cohort study. Psychol Med. 2013 Aug;43(8):1773-83.

Huang W, Wang G, Lu SE, Kipen H, Wang Y, Hu M, Lin W, Rich D, Ohman-Strickland P, Diehl SR, Zhu P, Tong J, Gong J, Zhu T, Zhang J. Inflammatory and oxidative stress responses of healthy young adults to changes in air quality during the Beijing Olympics. Am J Respir Crit Care Med. 2012 Dec 1;186(11):1150-9.

Alanna Morris, Dorothy Coverson, Lucy Fike, Yusuf Ahmed, Neli Stoyanova, W. Craig Hooper, Gary Gibbons, Donald Bliwise, Viola Vaccarino, Rebecca Din-Dzietham, Arshed Quyyumi. Sleep Quality and Duration are Associated with Higher Levels of Inflammatory Biomarkers: the META-Health Study. Circulation, 23 November 2010; 122: A17806.

Cassidy A, Rogers G, Peterson JJ, Dwyer JT, Lin H, Jacques PF. Higher dietary anthocyanin and flavonol intakes are associated with anti-inflammatory effects in a population of US adults. Am J Clin Nutr. 2015 Jul;102(1):172-81.

Shilpa N Bhupathiraju and Katherine L Tucker. Greater variety in fruit and vegetable intake is associated with lower inflammation in Puerto Rican adults. Am J Clin Nutr. 2011 January; 93(1): 37–46.

Esmaillzadeh A, Azadbakht L. Home use of vegetable oils, markers of systemic inflammation, and endothelial dysfunction among women. Am J Clin Nutr. 2008 Oct;88(4):913-21.

Tushar Singh, MD, MS, Anne B. Newman, MD, MPH. Inflammatory markers in population studies of aging. Ageing Res Rev. 2011 July; 10(3): 319–329.

Lorente-Cebrián S, Costa AG, Navas-Carretero S, Zabala M, Laiglesia LM, Martínez JA, Moreno-Aliaga MJ. An update on the role of omega-3 fatty acids on inflammatory and degenerative diseases. J Physiol Biochem. 2015 Jun;71(2):341-9.

Bogna Grygiel-Górniak,, Mariusz Puszczewicz Fatigue and interleukin-6 – a multi-faceted relationship. Reumatologia. 2015; 53(4): 207-212.

Cavicchia PP, Steck SE, Hurley TG, Hussey JR, Ma Y, Ockene IS, Hébert JR. A new dietary inflammatory index predicts interval changes in serum high-sensitivity C-reactive protein. J Nutr. 2009 Dec;139(12):2365-72.

1119. Rosenkranz MA, Davidson RJ, Maccoon DG, Sheridan JF, Kalin NH, Lutz A. A comparison of mindfulness-based stress reduction and an active control in modulation of neurogenic inflammation. Brain Behav Immun. 2013 Jan;27(1):174-84.

Bonaz B, Sinniger V, Pellissier S. Anti-inflammatory properties of the vagus nerve: potential therapeutic implications of vagus nerve stimulation. J Physiol. 2016 Apr 5.

Bhasin MK, Dusek JA, Chang BH, Joseph MG, Denninger JW, Fricchione GL, Benson H, Libermann TA. Relaxation response induces temporal transcriptome changes in energy metabolism, insulin secretion and inflammatory pathways. PLoS One. 2013 May 1;8(5):e62817.

Black DS, Cole SW, Irwin MR, Breen E, St Cyr NM, Nazarian N, Khalsa DS, Lavretsky H. Yogic meditation reverses NF-κB and IRF-related transcriptome dynamics in leukocytes of family dementia caregivers in a randomized controlled trial. Psychoneuroendocrinology. 2013 Mar;38(3):348-55.

PHYSICAL EXERCISE

Moore SC, Patel AV, Matthews CE, Berrington de Gonzalez A, Park Y, Katki HA, Linet MS, Weiderpass E, Visvanathan K, Helzlsouer KJ, Thun M, Gapstur SM, Hartge P, Lee IM. Leisure time physical activity of moderate to vigorous intensity and mortality: a large pooled cohort analysis. PLoS Med. 2012;9(11):e1001335.

Karstoft K, Pedersen BK. Skeletal muscle as a gene regulatory endocrine organ. Curr Opin Clin Nutr Metab Care. 2016 Jul;19(4):270-5.

Crane JD, MacNeil LG, Lally JS, Ford RJ, Bujak AL, Brar IK, Kemp BE, Raha S, Steinberg GR, Tarnopolsky MA. Exercise-stimulated interleukin-15 is controlled by AMPK and regulates skin metabolism and aging. Aging Cell. 2015 Aug;14(4):625-34.

Saeid Golbidi, Mohammad Badran, and Ismail Laher. Antioxidant and Anti-Inflammatory Effects of Exercise in Diabetic Patients. Exp Diabetes Res. 2012: 941868

Zoladz JA, Pilc A. The effect of physical activity on the brain derived neurotrophic factor: from animal to human studies. J Physiol Pharmacol. 2010 Oct;61(5):533-41.

Pieramico V, Esposito R, Sensi F, Cilli F, Mantini D, Mattei PA, Frazzini V, Ciavardelli D, Gatta V, Ferretti A, Romani GL, Sensi SL. Combination training in aging individuals modifies functional connectivity and cognition, and is potentially affected by dopamine-related genes. PLoS One. 2012;7(8):e43901.

Dipietro L, Gribok A, Stevens MS, Hamm LF, Rumpler W. Three 15-min Bouts of Moderate Postmeal Walking Significantly Improves 24-h Glycemic Control in Older People at Risk for Impaired Glucose Tolerance. Diabetes Care. 2013 Oct;36(10):3262-8.

SLEEP

Jane E Ferrie, Martin J Shipley, Tasnime N Akbaraly, Michael G Marmot, M Kivimäki, Archana Singh-Manoux. Change in Sleep Duration and Cognitive Function: Findings from the Whitehall II Study. Sleep. 2011;34 pp 565-573.

John Axelsson, Tina Sundelin, Michael Ingre, Eus J W Van Someren, Andreas Olsson, Mats Lekander. Beauty sleep: experimental study on the perceived health and attractiveness of sleep deprived people. BMJ Dec 14;341:c6614

89. Gozal D. Sleep, sleep disorders and inflammation in children.Sleep Med. 2009 Sep;10 Suppl 1:S12-6

Irwin MR, Olmstead R, Carroll JE. Sleep Disturbance, Sleep Duration, and Inflammation: A Systematic Review and Meta-Analysis of Cohort Studies and Experimental Sleep Deprivation. Biol Psychiatry. 2015 Jun 1. pii: S0006-3223(15)00437-0.

Carroll JE, Cole SW, Seeman TE, Breen EC, Witarama T, Arevalo JM, Ma J5, Irwin MR.

Partial sleep deprivation activates the DNA damage response (DDR) and the senescence-associated secretory phenotype (SASP) in aged adult humans. Brain Behav Immun. 2016 Jan;51:223-9.

Xie L, Kang H, Xu Q, Chen MJ, Liao Y, Thiyagarajan M, O'Donnell J, Christensen DJ, Nicholson C, Iliff JJ, Takano T, Deane R, Nedergaard M. Sleep drives metabolite clearance from the adult brain. Science. 2013 Oct 18;342(6156):373-7.

INTESTINAL FLORA

Michael A. Conlon, Anthony R. Bird. The Impact of Diet and Lifestyle on Gut Microbiota and Human Health Nutrients. 2015 Jan; 7(1): 17–44.

Joanne Slavin. Fiber and Prebiotics: Mechanisms and Health Benefits. Nutrients. 2013 Apr; 5(4): 1417–1435.

Thomas LV, Ockhuizen T, Suzuki K. Exploring the influence of the gut microbiota and probiotics on health: a symposium report. Br J Nutr. 2014 Jul;112 Suppl 1:S1-18.

1754. Freedberg DE, Lebwohl B, Abrams JA. The impact of proton pump inhibitors on the human gastrointestinal microbiome. Clin Lab Med. 2014 Dec;34(4):771-85.

Peguet-Navarro J, Dezutter-Dambuyant C, Buetler T, Leclaire J, Smola H, Blum S, Bastien P, Breton L, Gueniche A. Supplementation with oral probiotic bacteria protects human cutaneous immune homeostasis after UV exposure-double blind, randomized, placebo controlled clinical trial. Eur J Dermatol. 2008 Sep-Oct;18(5):504-11.

Erdman SE, Poutahidis T. Probiotic 'glow of health': it's more than skin deep. Benef Microbes. 2014 Jun 1;5(2):109-19. doi: 10.3920/BM2013.0042.

Galland L. The gut microbiome and the brain. J Med Food. 2014 Dec;17(12):1261-72.

Kellow NJ, Coughlan MT, Savige GS, Reid CM. Effect of dietary prebiotic supplementation on advanced glycation, insulin resistance and inflammatory biomarkers in adults with pre-diabetes: a study protocol for a double-blind placebo-controlled randomised crossover clinical trial. BMC Endocr Disord. 2014 Jul 10;14:55.

TELOMERES

Shammas MA. Telomeres, lifestyle, cancer, and aging. Curr Opin Clin Nutr Metab Care. 2011 Jan;14(1):28-34.

Honig LS, Kang MS, Schupf N, Lee JH, Mayeux R. Association of Shorter Leukocyte Telomere Repeat Length With Dementia and Mortality. Arch Neurol. 2012 Jul 23:1-8.

Saßenroth D, Meyer A, Salewsky B, Kroh M, Norman K, Steinhagen-Thiessen E, Demuth ISports and Exercise at Different Ages and Leukocyte Telomere Length in Later Life - Data from the Berlin Aging Study II (BASE-II). PLoS One. 2015 Dec 2;10(12):e0142131.

Njajou OT, Hsueh WC, Blackburn EH, Newman AB, Wu SH, Li R, Simonsick EM, Harris TM, Cummings SR, Cawthon RM; Health ABC study. Association between telomere length, specific causes of death, and years of healthy life in health, aging, and body composition, a population-based cohort study. J Gerontol A Biol Sci Med Sci. 2009 Aug;64(8):860-4.

Effros RB. Telomere/telomerase dynamics within the human immune system: effect of chronic infection and stress. Exp Gerontol. 2011 Feb-Mar;46(2-3):135-40.

Jeon HS, Choi JE, Jung DK, Choi YY, Kang HG, Lee WK, Yoo SS, Lim JO, Park JY. Telomerase activity and the risk of lung cancer. J Korean Med Sci. 2012 Feb;27(2):141-5. Epub 2012 Jan 27.

Leung CW, Laraia BA, Needham BL, Rehkopf DH, Adler NE, Lin J, Blackburn EH, Epel ES. Soda and cell aging: associations between sugar-sweetened beverage consumption and leukocyte telomere length in healthy adults from the National Health and Nutrition Examination Surveys. Am J Public Health. 2014 Dec;104(12):2425-31.

Brydon L, Lin J, Butcher L, Hamer M, Erusalimsky JD, Blackburn EH, Steptoe A. Hostility and cellular aging in men from the Whitehall II cohort. Biol Psychiatry. 2012 May 1;71(9):767-73.

Entringer S, Epel ES, Kumsta R, Lin J, Hellhammer DH, Blackburn EH, Wüst S, Wadhwa PD. Stress exposure in intrauterine life is associated with shorter telomere length in young adulthood. Proc Natl Acad Sci USA 2011 Aug 16;108(33):E513-8.

Puterman E, Lin J, Krauss J, Blackburn EH, Epel ES. Determinants of telomere attrition over 1 year in healthy older women: stress and health behaviors matter. Mol Psychiatry. Mol Psychiatry. 2015 Apr;20(4):529-35.

Ornish D, Lin J, Daubenmier J, Weidner G, Epel E, Kemp C, Magbanua MJ, Marlin R, Yglecias L, Carroll PR, Blackburn EH. Increased telomerase activity and comprehensive lifestyle changes: a pilot study. Lancet Oncol. 2008 Nov;9(11):1048-57.

Ornish D, Lin J, Chan JM, Epel E, Kemp C, Weidner G, Marlin R, Frenda SJ, Magbanua MJ, Daubenmier J, Estay I, Hills NK, Chainani-Wu N, Carroll PR,Blackburn EH. Effect of comprehensive lifestyle changes on telomerase activity and telomere length in men with biopsy-proven low-risk prostate cancer: 5-year follow-up of a descriptive pilot study. Lancet Oncol. 2013 Oct;14(11):1112-20.

Daubenmier J, Lin J, Blackburn E, Hecht FM, Kristeller J, Maninger N, Kuwata M, Bacchetti P, Havel PJ, Epel E. Changes in stress, eating, and metabolic factors are related to changes in telomerase activity in a randomized mindfulness intervention pilot study. Psychoneuroendocrinology. 2012 Jul;37(7):917-28.

Zvereva MI, Shcherbakova DM, Dontsova OA. Telomerase: structure, functions, and activity regulation. Biochemistry (Mosc). 2010 Dec;75(13):1563-83.

Wang XB, Zhu L, Huang J, Yin YG, Kong XQ, Rong QF, Shi AW, Cao KJ. Resveratrol-induced augmentation of telomerase activity delays senescence of endothelial progenitor cells. Chin Med J (Engl). 2011 Dec;124(24):4310-5.

Vera E, Bernardes de Jesus B, Foronda M, Flores JM, Blasco MA. Telomerase reverse transcriptase synergizes with calorie restriction to increase health span and extend mouse longevity. PLoS One. 2013;8(1):e53760.

GLYCATION

Palimeri S, Palioura E, Diamanti-Kandarakis E. Current perspectives on the health risks associated with the consumption of advanced glycation end products: recommendations for dietary management. Diabetes Metab Syndr Obes. 2015 Sep 1;8:415-26.

Clarke RE, Dordevic AL, Tan SM, Ryan L, Coughlan MT. Dietary Advanced Glycation End Products and Risk Factors for Chronic Disease: A Systematic Review of Randomised Controlled Trials. Nutrients. 2016 Mar 1;8(3):125.

Nguyen HP, Katta R. Sugar Sag: Glycation and the Role of Diet in Aging Skin. Skin Therapy Lett. 2015 Nov;20(6):1-5.

Semba RD, Nicklett EJ, Ferrucci L. Does accumulation of advanced glycation end products contribute to the aging phenotype? J Gerontol A Biol Sci Med Sci. 2010 Sep;65(9):963-75.

Sell DR, Monnier VM. Molecular basis of arterial stiffening: role of glycation - a mini-review. Gerontology. 2012;58(3):227-37.

Elosta A, Ghous T, Ahmed N. Natural products as anti-glycation agents: possible therapeutic potential for diabetic complications. Curr Diabetes Rev. 2012 Mar;8(2):92-108.

Claudia Luevano-Contreras, Karen Chapman-Novakofski. Dietary Advanced Glycation End Products and Aging. Nutrients. 2010 December; 2(12): 1247-1265.

Yamagishi S. Role of advanced glycation end products (AGEs) in osteoporosis in diabetes. Curr Drug Targets. 2011 Dec;12(14):2096-102.

Uchiki T, Weikel KA, Jiao W, Shang F, Caceres A, Pawlak D, Handa JT, Brownlee M, Nagaraj R, Taylor A. Glycation-altered proteolysis as a pathobiologic mechanism that links dietary glycemic index, aging, and age-related disease (in nondiabetics). Aging Cell. 2012 Feb;11(1):1-13.

Cai W, Uribarri J, Zhu L, Chen X, Swamy S, Zhao Z, Grosjean F, Simonaro C, Kuchel GA, Schnaider-Beeri M, Woodward M, Striker GE, Vlassara H. Oral glycotoxins are a modifiable cause of dementia and the metabolic syndrome in mice and humans. Proc Natl Acad Sci U S A. 2014 Apr 1;111(13):4940-5.

Sun K, Semba RD, Fried LP, Schaumberg DA, Ferrucci L, Varadhan R. Elevated Serum Carboxymethyl-Lysine, an Advanced Glycation End Product, Predicts Severe Walking Disability in Older Women: The Women's Health and Aging Study I. J Aging Res. 2012;2012:586385.

Elsamma Chacko Blunting post-meal glucose surges in people with diabetes. World J Diabetes. 2016 Jun 10; 7(11): 239-242.

Goto A, Noda M, Sawada N, Kato M, Hidaka A, Mizoue T, Shimazu T, Yamaji T, Iwasaki M, Sasazuki S, Inoue M, Kadowaki T, Tsugane S;JPHC Study Group. High hemoglobin A1c levels within the non-diabetic range are associated with the risk of all cancers. Int J Cancer. 2016 Apr 1;138(7):1741-53.

Mitrou P, Petsiou E, Papakonstantinou E, Maratou E, Lambadiari V, Dimitriadis P, Spanoudi F, Raptis SA, Dimitriadis G. Vinegar Consumption Increases Insulin-Stimulated Glucose Uptake by the Forearm Muscle in Humans with Type 2 Diabetes. J Diabetes Res. 2015;2015:175204.

Handunge Kumudu Irani Perera, Charith Sandaruwan Handuwalage Analysis of glycation induced protein cross-linking inhibitory effects of some antidiabetic plants and spices. BMC Complement Altern Med. 2015; 15: 175.

Dearlove RP, Greenspan P, Hartle DK, Swanson RB, Hargrove JL. Inhibition of protein glycation by extracts of culinary herbs and spices. J Med Food. 2008 Jun;11(2):275-81.

Sotiria Palimeri, Eleni Palioura, Evanthia Diamanti-Kandarakis Current perspectives on the health risks associated with the consumption of advanced glycation end products: recommendations for dietary management. Diabetes Metab Syndr Obes. 2015; 8: 415-426.

Liatis S, Grammatikou S, Poulia KA, Perrea D, Makrilakis K, Diakoumopoulou E, Katsilambros N. Vinegar reduces postprandial hyperglycaemia in patients with type II diabetes when added to a high, but not to a low, glycaemic index meal.Eur J Clin Nutr. 2010 Jul;64(7):727-32.

Ostman E, Granfeldt Y, Persson L, Björck I. Vinegar supplementation lowers glucose and insulin responses and increases satiety after a bread meal in healthy subjects. Eur J Clin Nutr. 2005 Sep;59(9):983-8.

Momma H, Niu K, Kobayashi Y, Guan L, Sato M, Guo H, Chujo M, Otomo A, Yufei C, Tadaura H, Saito T, Mori T, Miyata T, Nagatomi R. Skin advanced glycation end product accumulation and muscle strength among adult men. Eur J Appl Physiol. 2011 Jul;111(7):1545-52.

Claudia Luevano-Contreras, Karen Chapman-Novakofski. Dietary Advanced Glycation End Products and Aging. Nutrients. 2010 December; 2(12): 1247-1265.

Uribarri J, Woodruff S, Goodman S, Cai W, Chen X, Pyzik R, Yong A, Striker GE, Vlassara H. Advanced glycation end products in foods and a practical guide to their reduction in the diet. J Am Diet Assoc. 2010 Jun;110(6):911-16.e12.

Saraswat M, Reddy PY, Muthenna P, Reddy GB. Prevention of non-enzymic glycation of proteins by dietary agents: prospects for alleviating diabetic complications. Br J Nutr. 2009 Jun;101(11):1714-21.

Dearlove RP, Greenspan P, Hartle DK, Swanson RB, Hargrove JL. Inhibition of protein glycation by extracts of culinary herbs and spices. J Med Food. 2008 Jun;11(2):275-81.

Perera HK, Handuwalage CS. Analysis of glycation induced protein cross-linking inhibitory effects of some antidiabetic plants and spices. BMC Complement Altern Med. 2015 Jun 9;15:175.

AUTOPHAGY

Madeo F, Zimmermann A, Maiuri MC, Kroemer G. Essential role for autophagy in life span extension. J Clin Invest. 2015 Jan;125(1):85-93.

Choi AM, Ryter SW, Levine B Autophagy in human health and disease. N Engl J Med. 2013 May 9;368(19):1845-6.

García-Prat L, Martínez-Vicente M, Perdiguero E, Ortet L, Rodríguez-Ubreva J, Rebollo E, Ruiz-Bonilla V, Gutarra S, Ballestar E, Serrano AL, Sandri M, Muñoz-Cánoves P. Autophagy maintains stemness by preventing senescence. Nature. 2016 Jan 7;529(7584):37-42.

Kiriyama Y, Nochi H. The Function of Autophagy in Neurodegenerative Diseases. Int J Mol Sci. 2015 Nov 9;16(11):26797-812.

Colman RJ, Anderson RM, Johnson SC, Kastman EK, Kosmatka KJ, Beasley TM, Allison DB, Cruzen C, Simmons HA, Kemnitz JW, Weindruch R. Caloric restriction delays disease onset and mortality in rhesus monkeys. Science. 2009 Jul 10;325(5937):201-4.

Makino N, Oyama J, Maeda T, Koyanagi M, Higuchi Y, Tsuchida K.Calorie restriction increases telomerase activity, enhances autophagy, and improves diastolic dysfunction in diabetic rat hearts. Mol Cell Biochem. 2015 May;403(1-2):1-11.

Stephen Anton, Christiaan Leeuwenburgh* Fasting or caloric restriction for Healthy Aging. Exp Gerontol. 2013 Oct; 48(10): 1003–1005.

Valter D. Longo, Mark P. Mattson. Fasting: Molecular Mechanisms and Clinical Applications. Cell Metab. 2014 Feb 4; 19(2): 181–192.

Zoe E. Gillespie, Joshua Pickering, Christopher H. Eskiw. Better Living through Chemistry: Caloric Restriction (CR) and CR Mimetics Alter Genome Function to Promote Increased Health and Lifespan. Front Genet. 2016; 7: 142.

Barger JL, Kayo T, Vann JM, Arias EB, Wang J, Hacker TA, Wang Y, Raederstorff D, Morrow JD, Leeuwenburgh C, et al. A low dose of dietary resveratrol partially mimics caloric restriction and retards aging parameters in mice. PLoS One. 2008 Jun 4; 3(6):e2264.

Benderdour M, Martel-Pelletier J, Pelletier JP, Kapoor M, Zunzunegui MV, Fahmi H1. Cellular Aging, Senescence and Autophagy Processes in Osteoarthritis. Curr Aging Sci. 2015;8(2):147-57.

Witte AV, Fobker M, Gellner R, Knecht S, Flöel A. Caloric restriction improves memory in elderly humans. Proc Natl Acad Sci U S A. 2009 Jan 27;106(4):1255-60.

Kirkland JL. Perspectives on cellular senescence and short term dietary restriction in adults. Aging (Albany NY). 2010 Sep;2(9):542-4.

Trepanowski JF, Canale RE, Marshall KE, Kabir MM, Bloomer RJ. Impact of caloric and dietary restriction regimens on markers of health and longevity in humans and animals: a summary of available findings. Nutr J. 2011 Oct 7;10:107.

Vera E, Bernardes de Jesus B, Foronda M, Flores JM, Blasco MA. Telomerase reverse transcriptase synergizes with calorie restriction to increase health span and extend mouse longevity. PLoS One. 2013;8(1):e53760.

Horne BD, May HT, Anderson JL, Kfoury AG, Bailey BM, McClure BS, Renlund DG, Lappé DL, Carlquist JF, Fisher PW, Pearson RR, Bair TL, Adams TD,Muhlestein JB; Intermountain Heart Collaborative Study.Usefulness of routine periodic fasting to lower risk of coronary artery disease in patients undergoing coronary angiography. Am J Cardiol. 2008 Oct 1;102(7):814-819.

Horne BD, Muhlestein JB, Lappé DL, May HT, Carlquist JF, Galenko O, Brunisholz KD, Anderson JL. Randomized cross-over trial of short-term water-only fasting: Metabolic and cardiovascular consequences. Nutr Metab Cardiovasc Dis. 2012 Dec 7. pii: S0939-4753(12)00257-8.

Frake RA, Ricketts T, Menzies FM, Rubinsztein DC. Autophagy and neurodegeneration. J Clin Invest. 2015 Jan;125(1):65-74.

Pallauf K, Rimbach G. Autophagy, polyphenols and healthy ageing. Ageing Res Rev. 2012 Apr 6;12(1):237-252.

Morselli E, Mariño G, Bennetzen MV, Eisenberg T, Megalou E, Schroeder S, Cabrera S, Bénit P, Rustin P, Criollo A, Kepp O, Galluzzi L, Shen S, Malik SA, Maiuri MC, Horio Y, López-Otín C, Andersen JS, Tavernarakis N, Madeo F, Kroemer G. Spermidine and resveratrol induce autophagy by distinct pathways converging on the acetylproteome.J Cell Biol. 2011 Feb 21;192(4):615-29.

Chang J, Wang Y, Shao L, Laberge RM, Demaria M, Campisi J, Janakiraman K, Sharpless NE, Ding S, Feng W, Luo Y, Wang X,Aykin-Burns N, Krager K, Ponnappan U, Hauer-Jensen M, Meng A, Zhou D. Clearance of senescent cells by ABT263 rejuvenates aged hematopoietic stem cells in mice. Nat Med. 2016 Jan;22(1):78-83.

Roos CM, Zhang B, Palmer AK, Ogrodnik MB, Pirtskhalava T, Thalji NM, Hagler M, Jurk D, Smith LA, Casaclang-Verzosa G, Zhu Y, Schafer MJ, Tchkonia T, Kirkland JL, Miller JD. Chronic senolytic treatment alleviates established vasomotor dysfunction in aged or atherosclerotic mice. Aging Cell. 2016 Oct;15(5):973-7.

Mendelsohn AR, Larrick JW. Rejuvenating Muscle Stem Cell Function: Restoring Quiescence and Overcoming Senescence. Rejuvenation Res. 2016 Apr;19(2):182-6.

Reut Yosef, Noam Pilpel, Ronit Tokarsky-Amiel, Anat Biran, Yossi Ovadya, Snir Cohen, Ezra Vadai, Liat Dassa, Elisheva Shahar, Reba Condiotti, Ittai Ben-Porath, Valery Krizhanovsky Directed elimination of senescent cells by inhibition of BCL-W and BCL-XL. Nat Commun. 2016; 7: 11190.

Malavolta M, Pierpaoli E, Giacconi R, Costarelli L, Piacenza F, Basso A, Cardelli M, Provinciali M. Pleiotropic Effects of Tocotrienols and Quercetin on Cellular Senescence: Introducing the Perspective of Senolytic Effects of Phytochemicals. Curr Drug Targets. 2016;17(4):447-59.

Baker DJ, Wijshake T, Tchkonia T, LeBrasseur NK, Childs BG, van de Sluis B, Kirkland JL, van Deursen JM. Clearance of p16Ink4a-positive senescent cells delays ageing-associated disorders. Nature. 2011 Nov 2;479(7372):232-6.

THE STRATEGY

Vaid M, Sharma SD, Katiyar SK. Proanthocyanidins inhibit photocarcinogenesis through enhancement of DNA repair and xeroderma pigmentosum group A-dependent mechanism. Cancer Prev Res (Phila). 2010 Dec;3(12):1621-9.

Meeran SM, Akhtar S, Katiyar SK. Inhibition of UVB-induced skin tumor development by drinking green tea polyphenols is mediated through DNA repair and subsequent inhibition of inflammation. J Invest Dermatol. 2009 May;129(5):1258-70.

Alleva R, Manzella N, Gaetani S, Ciarapica V, Bracci M, Caboni MF, Pasini F, Monaco F, Amati M, Borghi B, Tomasetti M. Organic honey supplementation reverses pesticide-induced genotoxicity by modulating dna damage response. Mol Nutr Food Res. 2016 Apr 30.

Silva JP, Gomes AC, Coutinho OP. Oxidative DNA damage protection and repair by polyphenolic compounds in PC12 cells. Eur J Pharmacol. 2008 Dec 28;601(1-3):50-60.

SKIN

Panich U, Sittithumcharee G, Rathviboon N, Jirawatnotai S. Ultraviolet Radiation-Induced Skin Aging: The Role of DNA Damage and Oxidative Stress in Epidermal Stem Cell Damage Mediated Skin Aging. Stem Cells Int. 2016;2016:7370642.

Purba MB, Kouris-Blazos A, Wattanapenpaiboon N, Lukito W, Rothenberg E, Steen B, Wahlqvist ML. Can skin wrinkling in a site that has received limited sun exposure be used as a marker of health status and biological age? Age Ageing. 2001 May;30(3):227-34.

Levkovich T, Poutahidis T, Smillie C, Varian BJ, Ibrahim YM, Lakritz JR, Alm EJ, Erdman SE. Probiotic bacteria induce a 'glow of health'. PLoS One. 2013;8(1):e53867.

Archer DF. Postmenopausal skin and estrogen. Gynecol Endocrinol. 2012 Oct;28 Suppl 2:2-6.

Smith RN, Mann NJ, Braue A, Mäkeläinen H, Varigos GA. A low-glycemic-load diet improves symptoms in acne vulgaris patients: a randomized controlled trial. Am J Clin Nutr. 2007 Jul;86(1):107-15.

Ying Chen, John Lyga. Brain-Skin Connection: Stress, Inflammation and Skin Aging. Inflamm Allergy Drug Targets. Jun 2014; 13(3): 177–190.

Williams S, Tamburic S, Lally C. Eating chocolate can significantly protect the skin from UV light. J Cosmet Dermatol. 2009 Sep;8(3):169-73.

Katiyar SK, Singh T, Prasad R, Sun Q, Vaid M. Epigenetic alterations in ultraviolet radiation-induced skin carcinogenesis: interaction of bioactive dietary components on epigenetic targets.Photochem Photobiol. 2012 Sep-Oct;88(5):1066-74.

Moehrle M, Dietrich H, Patz CD, Häfner HM. Sun protection by red wine? J Dtsch Dermatol Ges. 2009 Jan;7(1):29-32, 29-33.

Chiang HM, Lin TJ, Chiu CY, Chang CW, Hsu KC, Fan PC, Wen KC. Coffea arabica extract and its constituents prevent photoaging by suppressing MMPs expression and MAP kinase pathway. Food Chem Toxicol. 2011 Jan;49(1):309-18.

Latreille J, Kesse-Guyot E, Malvy D, Andreeva V, Galan P, Tschachler E, Hercberg S, Guinot C, Ezzedine K.Association between dietary intake of n-3 polyunsaturated fatty acids and severity of skin photoaging in a middle-aged Caucasian population. J Dermatol Sci. 2013 Jul 23. pii: S0923-1811(13)00250-8.

Vierkötter A, Schikowski T, Ranft U, Sugiri D, Matsui M, Krämer U, Krutmann J. Airborne particle exposure and extrinsic skin aging. J Invest Dermatol. 2010 Dec;130(12):2719-26.

Martires KJ, Fu P, Polster AM, Cooper KD, Baron ED. Factors that affect skin aging: a cohort-based survey on twins. Arch Dermatol. 2009 Dec;145(12):1375-9.

Accorsi-Neto A, Haidar M, Simões R, Simões M, Soares-Jr J, Baracat E. Effects of isoflavones on the skin of postmenopausal women: a pilot study. Clinics (Sao Paulo). 2009;64(6):505-10.

Izumi T, Saito M, Obata A, Arii M, Yamaguchi H, Matsuyama A. Oral intake of soy isoflavone aglycone improves the aged skin of adult women. J Nutr Sci Vitaminol (Tokyo). 2007 Feb;53(1):57-62.

Lipovac M, Chedraui P, Gruenhut C, Gocan A, Kurz C, Neuber B, Imhof M. Effect of Red Clover Isoflavones over Skin, Appendages, and Mucosal Status in Postmenopausal Women. Obstet Gynecol Int. 2011;2011:949302.

Peguet-Navarro J, Dezutter-Dambuyant C, Buetler T, Leclaire J, Smola H, Blum S, Bastien P, Breton L, Gueniche A. Supplementation with oral probiotic bacteria protects human cutaneous immune homeostasis after UV exposure-double blind, randomized, placebo controlled clinical trial. Eur J Dermatol. 2008 Sep-Oct;18(5):504-11.

Bhattacharyya TK, Merz M, Thomas JR. Modulation of cutaneous aging with calorie restriction in Fischer 344 rats: a histological study. Arch Facial Plast Surg. 2005 Jan-Feb;7(1):12-6.

ABOUT THE AUTHOR

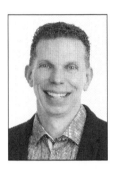

DR. DANIEL MINIER is a dermatologist who has been affiliated with the University of Sherbrooke for 20 years. Although patient care is his major focus, some of his time is devoted to supervising medical students and residents and engaging in clinical research projects.

He is also a Fellow of the American Academy of Dermatology and of the Royal College of Physicians of Canada. Moreover, he is an examination board member for the Royal College of Physicians of Canada. As a dermatologist, he is ideally placed to witness inequalities in the aging process. His book offers solutions to this problem for our society, which must prepare for what appears to be an ever-lengthening life expectancy. Daniel and his family live in Quebec.